Living Better with ASTHMA

A Doctor's Practical Guide to Asthma Control

Dr Prabhat Das

MD, PhD, FACP

Better Health with Dr Das Series

Hardcover ISBN: 978-1-971672-46-5

Paperback ISBN: 978-1-971672-45-8

eBook ISBN: 978-1-971672-44-1

Printed in the United States of America

Table of Content:

Disclaimer

This book is intended solely for educational and informational purposes. It is not meant to replace personal medical advice, diagnosis, or treatment.

Although I am a licensed physician, reading this book does not establish a doctor-patient relationship. Each individual's health condition, medical history, and risk factors are unique. Any medical decision should be made in partnership with your own healthcare professional who understands your specific situation.

Medical science is continually advancing. New research and updated guidelines may lead to changes in recommendations over time.

About the Author

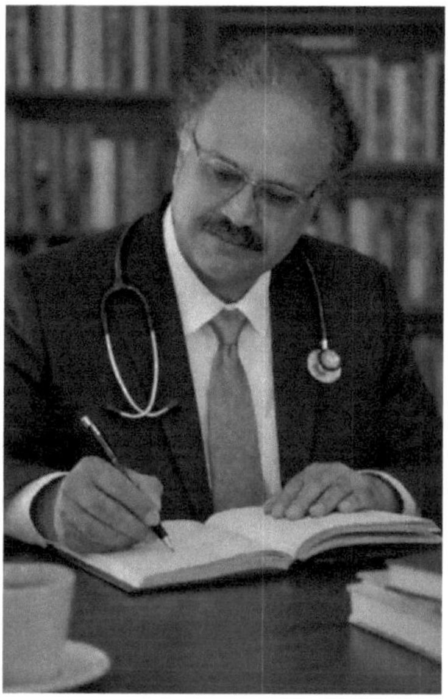

I am Dr Prabhat Das, MD, PhD, FACP. My journey in medicine began in India and, over the past thirty-five years, has continued in the United States, where I have had the privilege of caring for patients across a wide range of medical settings. I am trained in Internal Medicine, Pulmonary Diseases, and Critical Care. For me, medicine has never been just a profession. It has been a lifelong commitment shaped by learning, service, and a deep respect for the trust patients place in their physician.

Over the years, I have had the honor of caring for patients in many different situations. I have seen individuals in my office for routine concerns, treated urgent conditions in busy emergency rooms, managed serious illnesses in the hospital, and cared for critically ill patients in intensive care units. Each setting has taught me something valuable. Each patient has added to my understanding of what it truly means to care for another human being.

But one lesson has stood above all others. Medicine is not only about tests, diagnoses, or treatments. It is about people. It is about listening carefully, understanding fears that are often left unspoken, and guiding patients through uncertainty with clarity and compassion. Again and again, I have seen that what people want most is simple, trustworthy information. They want to understand what is happening in their bodies. They want to feel confident about the decisions they are making for their health and for their families.

These experiences have deeply shaped how I think about health, illness, prevention, and the human side of healing.

That is the reason behind the '**Better Health with Dr Das Series'**. Through these books, I hope to reach individuals I may never meet in person but who are searching for clear and reliable guidance. In today's world, health information is everywhere, yet much of it is confusing, overwhelming, and sometimes misleading. My goal is to cut through that noise and present important medical topics in a way that is simple, practical, and reassuring.

Every page of this series is guided by two foundations: reliable scientific knowledge and decades of real-world clinical experience. I want you, the reader, to feel informed, confident, and empowered. Not overwhelmed. Not confused. But clear about what you can do, step by step, to improve your health.

If even one reader feels less anxious, more informed, or better prepared to take control of their health after reading these books, then this work has served its purpose.

Helping people live healthier, longer, more confident and better-informed lives remains one of the greatest privileges of my life.

INTRODUCTION

If you are reading this book, asthma has likely touched your life in some way.

Perhaps you have recently been diagnosed and are trying to make sense of a condition that still feels unfamiliar.

Perhaps you have lived with asthma for years, yet still have questions.

Perhaps you are reading for a child, a spouse, a parent, or someone you love.

Whatever brings you here, welcome.

You are not alone.

Asthma is common. Yet it is often misunderstood.

Many people think asthma means only occasional wheezing or sudden breathing attacks. But asthma is often more complex than that. It can raise questions about symptoms, triggers, medicines, activity, sleep, uncertainty, and sometimes fear.

Those questions are real.

And they deserve clear, honest answers.

That is why I wrote this book.

As a physician, I have seen something repeatedly over many years of caring for patients:

People often do better when they understand their condition.

Understanding reduces fear.

Understanding improves decisions.

Understanding helps people ask better questions.

And better questions often lead to better care.

That belief runs through every page of this book.

This is not a technical textbook.

It is not written for specialists.

And it is not meant to overwhelm you.

It is a practical guide written in plain language, designed to help you understand asthma more clearly, think more confidently, and participate more actively in your care.

You do not need a medical background to read it.

Only curiosity.

And perhaps a willingness to look at asthma with fresh eyes.

This book begins with the basics.

What asthma is.

Why it may develop.

How symptoms may appear.

How asthma is diagnosed.

From there, we move step by step into triggers, treatment, inhalers, monitoring, flare-ups, living actively, difficult-to-control asthma, newer treatments, special situations, and the future of asthma care.

Later chapters focus on long-term living, common questions, and what I hope you carry forward from the book as a whole.

The book is designed to build understanding gradually.

Step by step.

You do not need to absorb everything at once.

Read it steadily.

Return to sections when questions arise.

Use it as a guide.

Use it as a reference.

Use it as a starting point for discussions with your physician.

That is part of its purpose.

I also want to say something important at the outset.

For many people, asthma can often be managed well.

That is worth saying clearly.

Because fear can easily outrun facts.

And I do not want fear setting the tone for this book.

I want understanding to set the tone.

And perspective.

And grounded hope.

That does not mean asthma should be taken lightly.

It should be respected.

But respect is different from fear.

And that distinction matters.

Very much.

If there is one message I hope runs through this entire book, it is this:

Asthma may require attention.

But it does not have to define the limits of your life.

I believe that.

And I hope this book helps you believe it too.

Thank you for allowing me to accompany you on this journey.

Let us begin.

CHAPTER 1: What Is Asthma? Understanding the Basics

Asthma is one of the most common chronic medical conditions in the world, yet it is often misunderstood.

Many people think asthma simply means occasional wheezing or sudden breathing attacks.

That is too narrow a view.

Asthma is much more than episodes of breathing difficulty.

At its core, asthma is a chronic condition involving the airways, the tubes that carry air in and out of the lungs.

When asthma is present, these airways may become overly sensitive and prone to inflammation. At times, the muscles around the airways may tighten, the airway lining may swell, and mucus may contribute to narrowing of the breathing passages. When this happens, airflow may become limited, and symptoms may develop.

That is the basic process.

And understanding that process matters.

Because asthma begins to make much more sense when you realize the problem is not simply attacks of symptoms, but what may be happening inside the airways.

That understanding is the foundation for everything that follows in this book.

What Happens in Asthma?

It may help to picture healthy airways as open, calm passages through which air moves freely.

In asthma, those airways may become irritated and overly reactive.

Three processes may contribute to symptoms:

Inflammation.

Airway narrowing.

And increased mucus.

Together, these changes may make breathing more difficult and may lead to symptoms such as cough, wheezing, chest tightness, or shortness of breath.

Sometimes symptoms may be mild.

Sometimes more serious.

Sometimes unpredictable.

That variability is one reason asthma can feel confusing.

But variability is often part of the condition itself.

What Is Asthma?

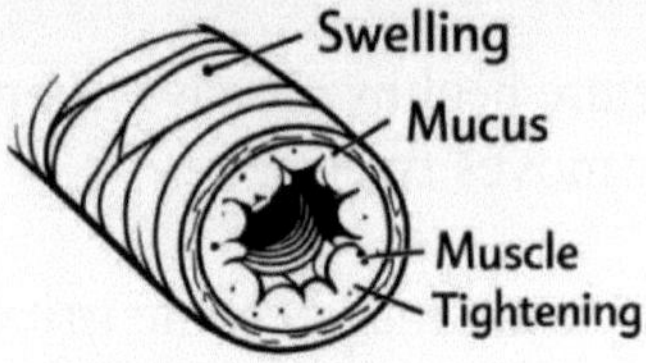

Inflamed Airways

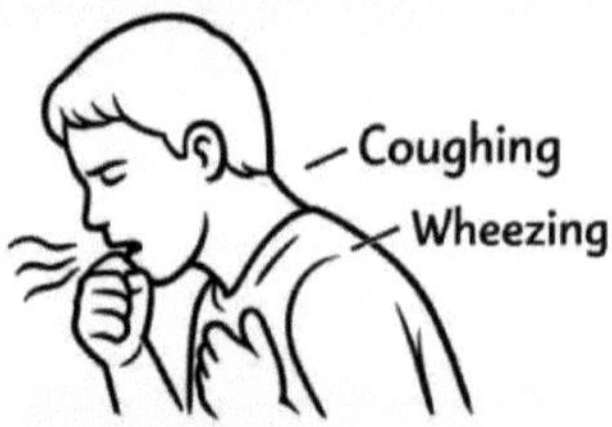

Breathing Difficulty

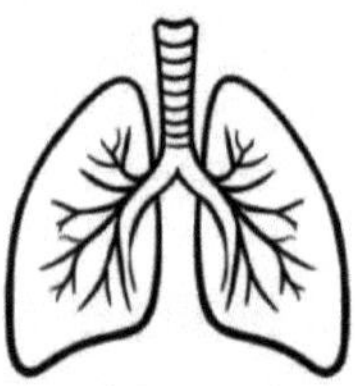

Asthma Symptoms

- Shortness of Breath
- Coughing
- Wheezing
- Chest Tightness

Why Do Symptoms Come and Go?

This is one of the first questions patients ask.

And it is a very good question.

If asthma is chronic, why can symptoms disappear for days, weeks, or even longer?

Because asthma is often dynamic.

Symptoms may increase when the airways are irritated or triggered.

And may improve when those influences settle.

That does not necessarily mean asthma has vanished.

And misunderstanding that can cause problems.

Asthma may be quiet.

And still matter.

That is important to understand.

Asthma Is Not the Same in Every Person

Another common misconception is that asthma looks the same in everyone.

It does not.

Some people have cough as the dominant symptom.

Some have wheezing.

Some notice symptoms mainly with exercise.

Others may have nighttime symptoms.

Patterns differ.

Triggers differ.

Severity differs.

And that is one reason asthma care often needs an individualized approach.

Chronic Does Not Mean Hopeless

When people hear the word chronic, they sometimes assume lifelong suffering.

Please do not make that assumption.

Chronic means ongoing.

It does not mean constant misery.

It does not mean you cannot do well.

And it does not mean good control is impossible.

Many people with asthma can achieve very good control.

What Asthma Is Not

Asthma is not weakness.

It is not nervousness.

It is not something to dismiss casually.

And it is not something patients should feel embarrassed about.

It is a real medical condition.

And it deserves thoughtful care.

Why Understanding Asthma Matters

Some readers may wonder:

Why spend time understanding disease?

Why not just discuss treatment?

Because understanding influences decisions.

And decisions influence outcomes.

Patients who understand asthma often recognize symptoms earlier, understand triggers better, use treatment more thoughtfully, and ask better questions.

Understanding is not separate from treatment.

It is part of good treatment.

A Word About Fear

Some readers may come to this book carrying fear.

Perhaps after a frightening episode.

Perhaps after years of uncertainty.

If so, I want to say this:

Understanding often reduces fear.

Because what is mysterious often feels more frightening than what is understood.

That is one reason education matters.

Doctor's Pearl

The first step toward managing asthma well is understanding that asthma is not simply episodes of symptoms.

It is a condition involving the airways.

And that understanding changes how everything else makes sense.

Myth vs Fact

Myth: If symptoms come and go, asthma cannot be a real chronic condition.

Fact: Asthma often varies.

Symptoms may come and go.

That variability may be part of the condition itself.

Common Mistakes to Avoid

Assuming asthma only matters when symptoms are severe.

Assuming feeling well means asthma has disappeared.

Thinking asthma is the same in every person.

Ignoring the importance of understanding the condition.

Red Flag Warnings

Seek prompt medical evaluation if:

- Breathing symptoms are severe or worsening
- Symptoms interfere with sleep or daily activities
- Breathing problems keep recurring
- You are uncertain whether symptoms may represent asthma or something else

Do not ignore serious breathing symptoms.

Key Points

- Asthma is a chronic condition involving the airways.
- Inflammation, airway narrowing, and mucus may contribute to symptoms.
- Symptoms may come and go, but asthma may still be present.
- Asthma does not look the same in every person.
- Chronic does not mean hopeless.
- Understanding asthma is the foundation of managing it well.

Chapter Summary

Asthma is often misunderstood.

But at its core, asthma is a chronic airway condition that may lead to breathing symptoms through inflammation and airway narrowing.

Symptoms may vary.

Patterns may differ.

And asthma may look different from person to person.

But one message should be clear:

Understanding asthma is the first step toward controlling it.

And that is where good asthma care begins.

Action Plan

- Begin thinking of asthma as a condition involving the airways, not simply isolated attacks.
- Reflect on how your symptoms have behaved over time.
- Notice whether symptoms seem to occur in patterns.
- Write down questions you have about asthma.
- Carry forward one important idea: understanding is part of treatment.

CHAPTER 2: What Causes Asthma? Risk Factors and Why Asthma Develops

One of the most common questions patients ask is simple:

Why did I develop asthma?

It is an understandable question.

And an important one.

But the answer is not always simple.

Because asthma usually does not arise from a single cause.

It often develops through a combination of influences.

Some inherited.

Some environmental.

Some not fully understood.

That uncertainty should be acknowledged.

Because honesty matters.

Medicine does not have every answer.

But we do know a great deal.

And what we do know can be helpful.

Asthma Often Develops Through More Than One Influence

Many people want one clear explanation.

One cause.

One reason.

But asthma is often more complicated than that.

It may develop through an interaction between biological tendencies and environmental exposures.

That means several factors may contribute at the same time.

And that is one reason asthma can look so different from person to person.

Genetics May Play a Role

Sometimes asthma appears to run in families.

That may matter.

If parents or close relatives have asthma, allergies, or related conditions, risk may sometimes be higher.

But genetics is not destiny.

And I want to emphasize that.

A family tendency does not guarantee asthma.

And people without a family history may still develop asthma.

That is important to understand.

Because genetic influence is often about susceptibility.

Not certainty.

Allergies and Asthma Are Often Linked

This is an important relationship.

Asthma and allergies may sometimes travel together.

Environmental allergens may contribute to airway irritation in some people.

And in some patients, this relationship may be important in understanding symptoms.

That is one reason allergies matter in asthma discussions.

Environmental Exposures May Matter

The air we breathe matters.

Sometimes greatly.

Environmental exposures may play a role in asthma development or worsening.

Examples may include irritants, pollution, smoke, occupational exposures, or other environmental influences.

The details vary.

And not every exposure affects every person the same way.

But environment matters.

And should not be overlooked.

Respiratory Infections May Sometimes Play a Role

This is another area patients often ask about.

Can infections contribute to asthma?

Sometimes they may be relevant.

And in some people, important.

Again, asthma is rarely one single story.

Often multiple influences may intersect.

Adult-Onset Asthma Can Happen

Some people assume asthma is mainly a childhood condition.

That is not correct.

Asthma may begin in adulthood.

And that surprises many people.

But it should not be dismissed.

If breathing symptoms develop later in life, thoughtful evaluation still matters.

Sometimes the Exact Cause Is Not Clear

Sometimes we cannot identify one precise reason a person developed asthma.

And that is true in medicine more often than people realize.

But uncertainty about one exact cause does not mean nothing is understood.

It simply means biology is often more complex than simple explanations suggest.

Risk Factors Are Not the Same as Blame

This is important.

Very important.

When discussing causes or risk factors, patients sometimes hear blame.

Please do not hear it that way.

Risk factors are not accusations.

They are ways of understanding possible influences.

That is very different.

Medicine should help patients understand.

Not judge them.

Why Understanding Causes Matters

If asthma already exists, why does understanding causes matter?

Because understanding influences prevention.

It may help identify exposures worth reducing.

Questions worth asking.

Patterns worth noticing.

And that may matter.

Understanding causes is not just about explaining the past.

It may help improve the future.

Doctor's Pearl

Asthma often develops through multiple influences rather than one single cause.

Understanding that can help you think about asthma more realistically.

Myth vs Fact

Myth: Asthma always has one clear cause.

Fact: Asthma often develops through multiple interacting influences, and sometimes no single cause can be identified.

Common Mistakes to Avoid

Assuming asthma must have one simple cause.

Assuming genetics means asthma was inevitable.

Ignoring possible environmental influences.

Confusing risk factors with blame.

Red Flag Warnings

Discuss further evaluation if:

- Breathing symptoms began recently and the cause seems unclear
- Workplace or environmental exposures may be relevant
- Allergies may be affecting symptoms
- You have questions about what may be contributing to your asthma

These are reasonable questions to raise.

Causes and Risk Factors of Asthma

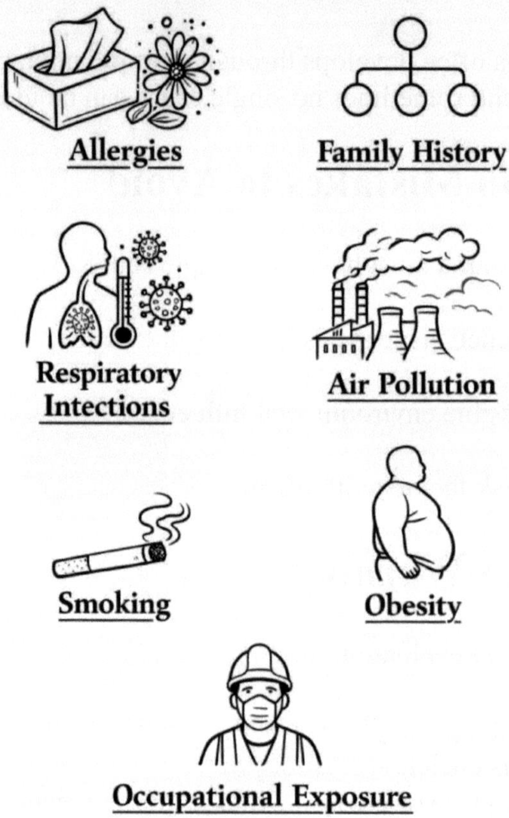

Key Points

- Asthma often develops through multiple influences.
- Genetics may contribute, but do not determine destiny.
- Allergies may sometimes be important.
- Environmental exposures may matter.
- Asthma may begin in adulthood.
- Sometimes no single exact cause can be identified.
- Understanding causes may help improve prevention and management.

Chapter Summary

Asthma often does not arise from one simple cause.

It may develop through a combination of inherited tendencies, environmental exposures, allergies, and other influences.

Sometimes the exact cause is not fully clear.

But understanding what may contribute to asthma can help patients think more clearly about prevention, triggers, and management.

Action Plan

- Think about whether asthma, allergies, or related conditions run in your family.
- Consider whether environmental exposures may be relevant in your life.
- Reflect on whether symptoms may have developed after certain changes or exposures.
- Write down questions you have about what may be contributing to your asthma.

- Carry forward one important idea: asthma often develops through multiple influences, not one simple cause.

CHAPTER 3: Recognizing Asthma: Signs and Symptoms

Asthma may announce itself clearly.

Or quietly.

Sometimes dramatically.

Sometimes subtly.

And that is one reason recognizing asthma is not always as straightforward as people assume.

Many people imagine asthma always looks the same.

A person wheezing.

Struggling visibly to breathe.

Having an obvious attack.

Sometimes that happens.

But not always.

And that misunderstanding can delay recognition.

Because asthma symptoms may sometimes be surprisingly varied.

That is why this chapter matters.

Recognizing asthma begins with recognizing patterns.

And patterns matter.

Cough May Be an Important Symptom

Many people do not think of cough as a possible asthma symptom.

But it may be.

And sometimes it may be a major clue.

Especially when cough keeps recurring.

Seems unexplained.

Or follows certain patterns.

Because repeated cough is sometimes dismissed too casually.

And it should not always be.

Wheezing

Wheezing is a symptom many people associate with asthma.

And understandably so.

It may be an important clue.

But it is important to understand something else.

Not every person with asthma wheezes.

And not every wheeze means asthma.

That distinction matters.

Because assumptions can mislead.

Shortness of Breath

Some patients describe a feeling of not getting enough air.

Others describe breathlessness with activity.

Or difficulty taking a satisfying breath.

Descriptions vary.

And that is normal.

Patients do not all experience symptoms the same way.

Nor describe them the same way.

Symptoms should be listened to carefully.

Not forced into rigid descriptions.

Chest Tightness

Some patients describe asthma not as wheezing at all.

But as tightness.

Pressure.

Constriction.

A sense that the chest feels closed.

That may matter.

Because symptoms do not always appear in textbook form.

Real life is often more varied than textbooks.

Nighttime Symptoms Matter

Symptoms that disturb sleep matter.

Repeated nighttime cough.

Wheezing.

Breathlessness.

These should not be dismissed casually.

They may be important clues.

And they deserve attention.

Symptoms May Follow Patterns

This is one of the most useful ideas in this chapter.

Patterns matter.

Sometimes more than isolated symptoms.

Symptoms after exercise.

Symptoms around exposures.

Symptoms at night.

Symptoms that recur in episodes.

Patterns may tell a story.

And often an important one.

Pay attention to patterns.

Because patterns may help bring clarity.

Symptoms May Come and Go

Symptoms may come and go.

And that variability sometimes confuses people.

They may think:

If symptoms disappear, maybe nothing is wrong.

Be careful.

That assumption may be mistaken.

Intermittent symptoms may still matter.

Very much.

Signs and Symptoms of Asthma

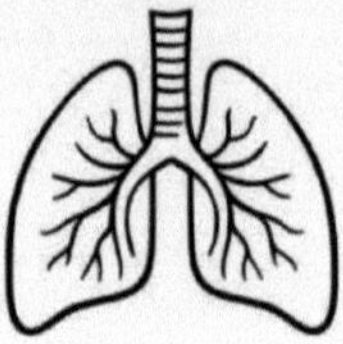

Shortness of Breath

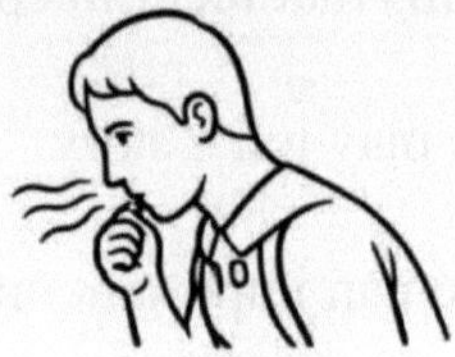

Coughing

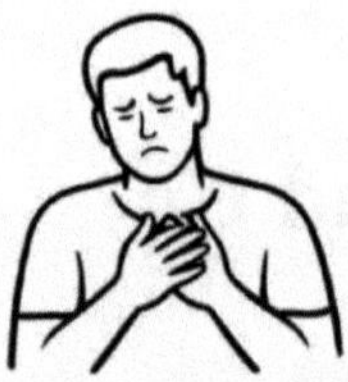

Chest Tightness

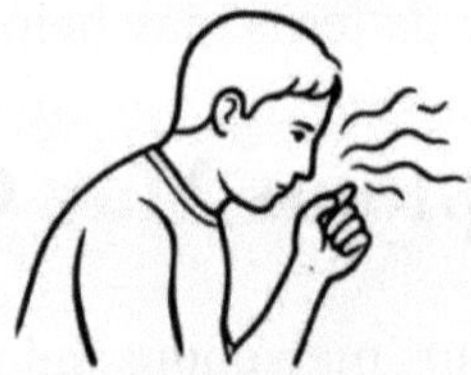

Wheezing

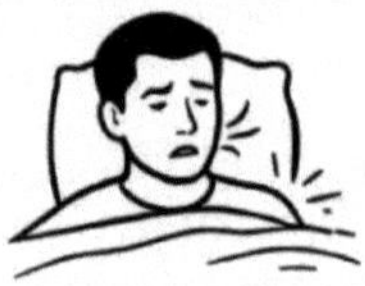

Nighttime Symptoms

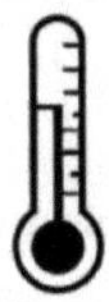

Increased Mucus

Mild Symptoms Should Not Always Be Ignored

Another common mistake is assuming only dramatic symptoms matter.

Not true.

Sometimes mild recurring symptoms deserve evaluation.

Especially when they keep returning.

Or seem unexplained.

Sometimes the quieter symptoms are the ones most easily missed.

And sometimes those are exactly the ones worth paying attention to.

Not Every Breathing Symptom Means Asthma

This is important too.

Because this chapter is about recognition.

Not self-diagnosis.

Breathing symptoms may have different causes.

And assumptions can be dangerous.

That is one reason proper evaluation matters.

And why the next chapter follows.

Because recognition is important.

But correct diagnosis is essential.

When Symptoms Seem Vague

Sometimes patients say:

I do not know how to describe it.

Something just feels off.

That matters too.

Do not dismiss vague but recurring symptoms simply because they are hard to describe.

Sometimes uncertainty itself deserves discussion.

That is reasonable.

Why Recognizing Symptoms Matters

Because recognition often comes before diagnosis.

And diagnosis often comes before better management.

That sequence matters.

Symptoms recognized early may lead to questions asked earlier.

Evaluation sought earlier.

And perhaps answers found earlier.

Doctor's Pearl

Asthma symptoms often reveal themselves through patterns.

Pay attention not only to symptoms, but to when they happen and how they recur.

That may matter greatly.

Myth vs Fact

Myth: Asthma always means obvious wheezing and dramatic breathing attacks.

Fact: Asthma symptoms may be varied, subtle, and sometimes easily overlooked.

Common Mistakes to Avoid

Assuming cough cannot be related to asthma.

Assuming no wheezing means no asthma.

Ignoring nighttime symptoms.

Dismissing mild recurring symptoms.

Assuming symptoms alone prove asthma without proper evaluation.

Red Flag Warnings

Seek prompt evaluation if:

- Breathing symptoms are worsening
- Symptoms disturb sleep
- Breathlessness limits activity
- Symptoms keep recurring without explanation
- Something about your breathing feels persistently abnormal

Do not ignore serious breathing symptoms.

Key Points

- Asthma symptoms may vary widely.
- Cough, wheezing, breathlessness, and chest tightness may all matter.
- Nighttime symptoms deserve attention.
- Patterns may be especially important.
- Symptoms may come and go.
- Mild recurring symptoms should not always be dismissed.
- Recognition is important, but proper diagnosis matters.

Chapter Summary

Recognizing asthma is not always as simple as people assume.

Symptoms may vary.

Patterns may differ.

And asthma may sometimes appear in subtle ways.

But one lesson should be clear:

Pay attention to symptoms.

Pay attention to patterns.

And do not dismiss recurring breathing concerns too casually.

Because recognition is often the first step toward answers.

Action Plan

- Reflect on whether you have noticed recurring breathing symptoms.
- Pay attention to patterns, including nighttime symptoms or exercise symptoms.
- Do not dismiss mild but repeated symptoms too quickly.
- Write down any breathing symptoms or patterns you want to understand better.
- Carry forward one important idea: symptoms often matter, but patterns may matter even more.

Transition to Chapter 4

Recognizing symptoms is important.

But another question follows naturally.

What if symptoms that seem like asthma are caused by something else?

That is where we turn next.

CHAPTER 4: Is It Really Asthma? Conditions That Can Mimic Asthma

One of the most important principles in medicine is simple:

Symptoms do not make a diagnosis.

That principle matters enormously.

Because breathing symptoms that seem like asthma are not always asthma.

And assuming otherwise can lead to mistakes.

Sometimes important mistakes.

That is why this chapter matters.

Recognizing asthma is important.

But recognizing that other conditions may resemble asthma is equally important.

This is where careful thinking matters.

And where assumptions can be dangerous.

Why This Question Matters

A person may have cough.

Wheezing.

Shortness of breath.

Chest tightness.

And naturally think:

This must be asthma.

Maybe.

But maybe not.

And that distinction matters.

Because treatment depends on getting the diagnosis right.

And getting the diagnosis right begins with considering alternatives.

That is not doubt.

That is good medicine.

Not Every Wheeze Means Asthma

This is one of the most common misunderstandings.

People hear wheezing and assume asthma.

Be careful.

Wheezing may occur in different conditions.

It is a clue.

Not a diagnosis.

And clues should lead to evaluation.

Not assumptions.

That is a very important distinction.

Chronic Obstructive Pulmonary Disease

Some breathing symptoms associated with asthma may also occur in Chronic Obstructive Pulmonary Disease.

These are different conditions.

And the distinction can matter greatly.

Especially because the right diagnosis influences the right treatment.

Vocal Cord Dysfunction and Similar Conditions

Some conditions involving the upper airway may sometimes resemble asthma.

That may surprise patients.

But it should not be ignored.

Because if something resembles asthma but is not asthma, recognizing that may change everything.

Sometimes dramatically.

Heart Conditions May Sometimes Cause Similar Symptoms

This is very important.

Because shortness of breath does not automatically mean lung disease.

Sometimes symptoms may relate to the heart.

And that possibility deserves respect.

Especially when symptoms do not fit a simple explanation.

Never assume.

Think broadly.

That is wise.

Acid Reflux May Sometimes Confuse the Picture

Sometimes symptoms may raise diagnostic questions.

And diagnostic questions deserve thoughtful evaluation.

That is the point.

Not to complicate things.

But to prevent oversimplification.

Anxiety-Related Breathing Symptoms

This requires careful handling.

And respect.

Breathing symptoms associated with anxiety or panic are real symptoms.

Real experiences.

They should never be dismissed.

But they may sometimes raise diagnostic questions.

And those questions deserve thoughtful evaluation.

That is very different from minimizing symptoms.

Sometimes More Than One Condition May Be Present

Sometimes the answer is not asthma or something else.

Sometimes it may be asthma and something else.

That layered possibility matters.

Because real medicine is sometimes more complicated than either-or thinking suggests.

Conditions That Mimic Asthma

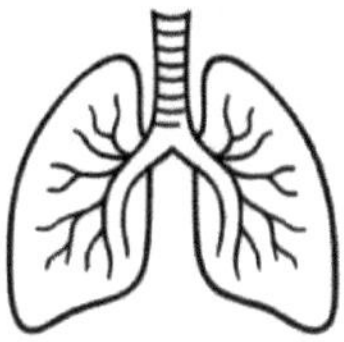

COPD

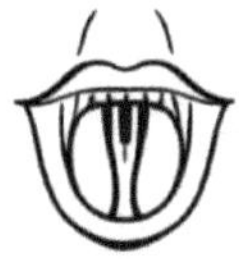

Vocal Cord Dysfunction

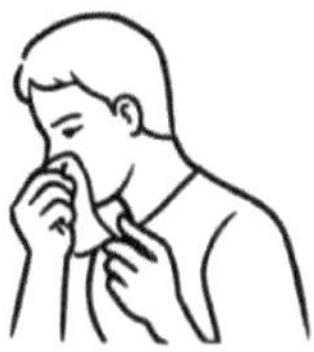

Allergic Rhinitis

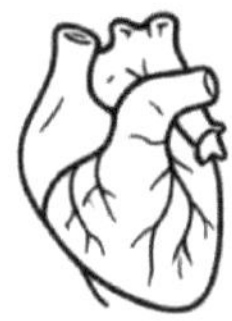

Heart Failure

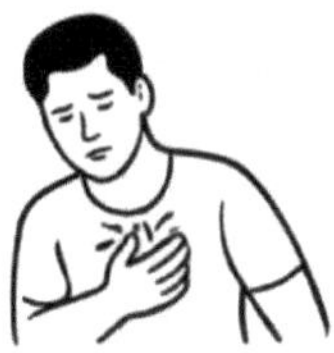

Acid Reflux

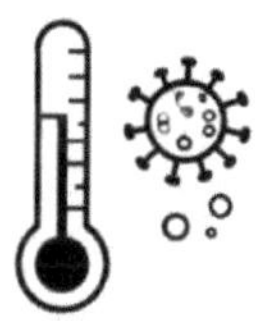

Respiratory Infections

Why Proper Testing Matters

Symptoms alone may suggest possibilities.

But they do not always establish the diagnosis.

And that is why testing matters.

And why the next chapter follows.

Because this chapter raises the question:

What else could this be?

And the next chapter addresses:

How do we sort that out?

Do Not Diagnose Yourself

This chapter is meant to encourage thoughtful evaluation.

Not self-diagnosis.

Please do not use symptom lists to diagnose yourself.

Or rule things in.

Or rule things out.

That is not the purpose here.

Why This Chapter Matters

Because assumptions can mislead.

Because symptoms may overlap.

Because not every breathing symptom means asthma.

And because the right diagnosis is the foundation of the right care.

Doctor's Pearl

Symptoms may provide clues.

But clues are not conclusions.

Good diagnosis requires thoughtful evaluation.

Never confuse the two.

Myth vs Fact

Myth: If I wheeze or feel short of breath, it must be asthma.

Fact: Several conditions may cause similar symptoms. Proper evaluation matters.

Common Mistakes to Avoid

Assuming breathing symptoms automatically mean asthma.

Assuming wheezing proves asthma.

Ignoring the possibility of other causes.

Trying to diagnose yourself based on symptoms alone.

Red Flag Warnings

Seek prompt evaluation if:

- Breathing symptoms are worsening
- Symptoms seem severe or unusual
- Treatment for presumed asthma does not seem to help
- Symptoms do not seem to fit a clear pattern
- Something about the diagnosis feels uncertain

These are important reasons to look deeper.

Key Points

- Symptoms alone do not make a diagnosis.
- Not every wheeze means asthma.
- Several conditions may mimic asthma.
- Sometimes more than one condition may be present.
- Proper evaluation and testing matter.
- The right diagnosis is the foundation of the right treatment.

Chapter Summary

Breathing symptoms that resemble asthma are not always caused by asthma.

And that is an important truth.

Several conditions may mimic asthma.

Sometimes closely.

That is why assumptions can be dangerous.

And why proper diagnosis matters so much.

Because the right diagnosis is where good care begins.

Action Plan

- If you have ever wondered whether symptoms could have another explanation, write down that question.
- Do not assume symptoms alone establish a diagnosis.
- If something about your symptoms or diagnosis feels unclear, raise that concern.
- Carry forward one important idea: similar symptoms do not always mean the same disease.
- Prepare for the next chapter, where we discuss how asthma is actually diagnosed.

Transition to Chapter 5

If symptoms alone do not establish the diagnosis, how is asthma diagnosed?

How do physicians sort it out?

That is where we turn next.

CHAPTER 5: How Asthma Is Diagnosed

By now, an important question naturally arises:

How is asthma actually diagnosed?

That is a very important question.

Because asthma is not diagnosed simply because someone coughs.

Or wheezes.

Or feels short of breath.

Symptoms matter.

But symptoms alone are not the whole story.

Diagnosis requires something more.

Thoughtful evaluation.

And often a combination of medical history, clinical judgment, physical examination, and testing.

Because the right diagnosis is the foundation of the right treatment.

And in medicine, foundations matter.

Diagnosis Often Begins With Listening

Patients sometimes assume diagnosis begins with machines.

Or tests.

Or numbers.

Sometimes it does not.

Often it begins with listening.

Careful listening.

Symptoms.

Patterns.

Timing.

Triggers.

Nighttime symptoms.

Exercise symptoms.

Past episodes.

All of these may matter.

Good diagnosis often begins there.

With the story.

Never underestimate the value of the story.

Medical History Matters

A thoughtful medical history may offer important clues.

Sometimes very important clues.

When symptoms occur.

How often they occur.

What seems to trigger them.

Whether symptoms come and go.

Whether symptoms worsen at night.

Whether allergies may be present.

Whether family history may be relevant.

These questions matter.

They may help shape diagnostic thinking.

Physical Examination May Matter Too

Physical examination may sometimes provide additional clues.

Sometimes subtle ones.

Sometimes important ones.

But I want to be honest.

A normal examination does not always rule out asthma.

And patients should understand that.

Because asthma may be variable.

And variability matters in diagnosis too.

Spirometry

One of the most important tests used in asthma evaluation is called spirometry.

Patients should at least know the name.

Because they may hear it often.

In simple terms, spirometry helps assess airflow.

And may help provide important information.

Because diagnosis is often stronger when symptoms and objective information are considered together.

Why Objective Testing Matters

Symptoms can sometimes mislead.

Not because patients are unreliable.

But because symptoms alone do not always distinguish one condition from another.

Objective testing may help bring clarity.

And clarity matters.

Especially when diagnoses may overlap.

Or uncertainty exists.

Sometimes Diagnosis Is Not Instant

Patients sometimes expect one visit.

One test.

One clear answer.

Sometimes that happens.

Sometimes it does not.

Sometimes diagnosis takes thoughtful follow-up.

Reassessment.

Further testing.

Time.

That should not be mistaken for failure.

Sometimes careful diagnosis takes time because careful medicine takes time.

When Diagnosis Is Uncertain

Uncertainty sometimes exists.

And honesty about uncertainty is part of good medicine.

If diagnosis is unclear, asking more questions.

Looking deeper.

Reassessing.

That is often not a problem.

That is often good care.

Never confuse uncertainty with incompetence.

Sometimes uncertainty is exactly what thoughtful medicine acknowledges honestly.

Why Response to Treatment Alone Is Not Enough

Some patients think:

If medicine seems to help, then it must be asthma.

Be careful.

That may oversimplify things.

Response to treatment may sometimes be informative.

But by itself, it may not settle everything.

Diagnosis should be approached thoughtfully.

Not casually.

How Is Asthma Diagnosed?

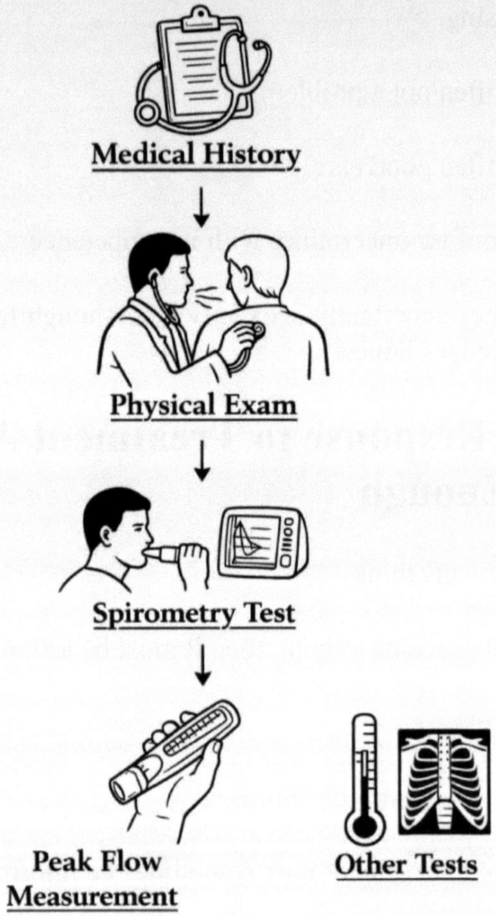

Diagnosis Is About Ruling Things In and Ruling Things Out

Diagnosis is often not simply proving one possibility.

It may also involve considering alternatives.

That connects directly with the previous chapter.

And it matters.

Because good diagnosis is often as much about avoiding the wrong conclusion as reaching the right one.

Do Not Be Discouraged If Testing Is Part of the Process

Some patients become anxious when testing is recommended.

Please do not assume testing means something alarming.

Often it simply means medicine is being careful.

And careful is good.

I would much rather see careful diagnosis than careless assumptions.

And patients should want that too.

Why This Chapter Matters

Because symptoms alone do not make a diagnosis.

Because proper evaluation matters.

Because testing may matter.

And because getting the diagnosis right may influence everything that follows.

Doctor's Pearl

Good asthma diagnosis often begins with symptoms and patterns.

But thoughtful diagnosis often goes beyond symptoms alone.

And that matters greatly.

Myth vs Fact

Myth: If I have symptoms that sound like asthma, the diagnosis is obvious.

Fact: Symptoms may raise suspicion, but proper diagnosis often requires careful evaluation and sometimes testing.

Common Mistakes to Avoid

Assuming symptoms alone prove asthma.

Assuming a normal examination rules out asthma.

Expecting diagnosis is always instant.

Confusing thoughtful testing with something alarming.

Red Flag Warnings

Discuss deeper evaluation if:

- Symptoms remain unexplained
- Diagnosis remains uncertain
- Presumed asthma treatment does not seem to help
- Symptoms seem inconsistent with the diagnosis
- You remain unclear about how the diagnosis was made

These are reasonable concerns to raise.

Key Points

- Asthma diagnosis often begins with careful listening and medical history.
- Physical examination may help, but may not tell the whole story.
- Spirometry may provide important information.
- Symptoms alone may not establish the diagnosis.
- Diagnosis may sometimes take time.
- Good diagnosis often includes considering alternative explanations.

Chapter Summary

Asthma diagnosis is not based on symptoms alone.

It often involves thoughtful evaluation.

Medical history.

Clinical judgment.

And sometimes testing such as spirometry.

Sometimes diagnosis is straightforward.

Sometimes it takes time.

But one lesson should be clear:

Getting the diagnosis right matters.

Because the right diagnosis is where the right treatment begins.

Action Plan

- Ask yourself whether you understand how the diagnosis was made.
- If you do not understand, ask.
- If testing such as spirometry has been discussed, learn why it matters.
- If uncertainty remains, do not hesitate to raise questions.
- Carry forward one important idea: good diagnosis is the foundation of good asthma care.

Transition to Chapter 6

Once asthma is diagnosed, the next question becomes:

What makes asthma worse?

And what may trigger symptoms?

That is where we turn next.

CHAPTER 6: Asthma Triggers: What Makes Symptoms Worse

Why do symptoms seem worse at certain times?

Why now and not yesterday?

Why in one place and not another?

Why after one activity but not another?

These are excellent questions.

And they lead to one of the most practical ideas in asthma management:

Triggers matter.

Because asthma symptoms do not always worsen randomly.

Sometimes something is provoking the airways.

And recognizing that may change everything.

Because understanding triggers may help reduce symptoms.

Reduce flare-ups.

And improve control.

That is powerful.

What Is a Trigger?

In simple terms, a trigger is something that may irritate the airways or contribute to worsening symptoms.

That is the broad idea.

And the practical idea is simple:

Some things may make asthma worse.

Recognizing those things matters.

Triggers May Differ From Person to Person

There is no universal trigger list that affects everyone the same way.

One person may react to one thing.

Another person may not.

That variability matters.

Because asthma is individualized.

And trigger patterns may be individualized too.

That is why observation matters.

Allergens May Matter in Some People

For some patients, allergens may play an important role.

And that deserves recognition.

The point is not to assume every allergen matters to every patient.

It is to understand that allergies may sometimes be relevant.

And if relevant, important.

Irritants May Trigger Symptoms

This is another important category.

Irritants may matter.

Smoke.

Strong odors.

Air pollution.

Chemical fumes.

Other irritants.

These may sometimes provoke symptoms.

Pay attention to what you notice.

That may be valuable.

Triggers for Asthma

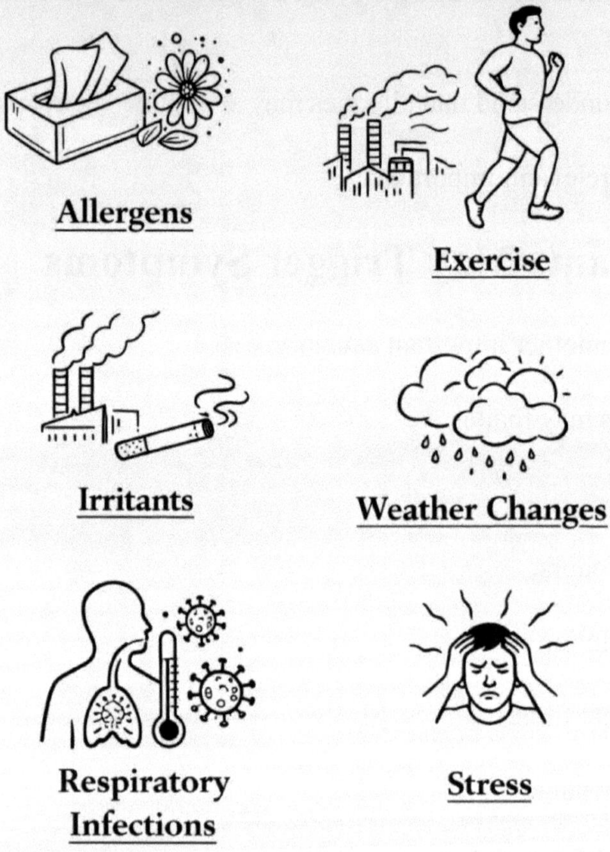

Respiratory Infections May Worsen Asthma

This is very important.

Because infections may sometimes trigger worsening.

Especially because respiratory infections are common.

And common things matter.

If symptoms worsen around infections, that may be important.

And worth recognizing.

Exercise May Trigger Symptoms in Some People

This often worries patients.

And it should be discussed carefully.

If exercise seems associated with symptoms, pay attention.

That does not automatically mean exercise should be abandoned.

We will discuss that more later.

But recognizing symptom patterns matters.

Weather and Environmental Conditions

Patients often notice this.

Cold air.

Seasonal changes.

Humidity.

Environmental shifts.

Sometimes symptoms seem affected.

Sometimes not.

But when patients notice patterns, they should pay attention.

Because observations may matter.

Emotional Stress May Sometimes Influence Symptoms

This requires balance.

Asthma is not simply emotional.

It is a real medical condition.

But life factors may sometimes affect symptoms or symptom experience.

That deserves thoughtful recognition.

Not oversimplification.

Sometimes There Is More Than One Trigger

Patients sometimes search for one trigger.

One cause.

One answer.

But sometimes there may be several.

And several may interact.

That matters.

Because real life is often more layered than simple explanations suggest.

Patterns Matter More Than Guessing

Do not rely on random guesses about triggers.

Look for patterns.

Repeated patterns.

Reliable patterns.

Those may be much more useful.

Patterns often teach more than assumptions.

Trigger Recognition Is About Awareness, Not Fear

I want to emphasize this.

Because I do not want readers becoming anxious about everything around them.

That is not the goal.

The goal is awareness.

Not hypervigilance.

Those are different things.

And the distinction matters.

Why Understanding Triggers Matters

Recognizing triggers may improve understanding and control.

This is not abstract knowledge.

This may affect daily life.

And that is why this chapter matters.

Doctor's Pearl

Pay attention not only to symptoms.

Pay attention to what seems to happen before symptoms.

That is often where trigger recognition begins.

Myth vs Fact

Myth: Asthma symptoms worsen randomly and cannot be understood.

Fact: Sometimes symptoms may reflect trigger patterns, and recognizing those patterns may help.

Common Mistakes to Avoid

Assuming everyone has the same triggers.

Assuming one trigger explains everything.

Guessing instead of looking for patterns.

Confusing awareness with fear.

Ignoring observations that may matter.

Red Flag Warnings

Discuss triggers more carefully if:

- Symptoms keep worsening without explanation
- Flare-ups seem linked to certain exposures
- Work or home environments may be affecting symptoms
- Infections repeatedly seem to worsen asthma
- You suspect patterns but do not understand them

These are excellent reasons to look more closely.

Key Points

- Triggers may worsen asthma symptoms.
- Triggers may differ from person to person.
- Allergens, irritants, infections, exercise, and environmental conditions may matter.
- Sometimes more than one trigger may be involved.
- Patterns often matter more than assumptions.
- Trigger awareness is about understanding, not fear.

Chapter Summary

Asthma symptoms do not always worsen randomly.

Sometimes triggers may be contributing.

And recognizing those triggers may improve understanding and control.

That is the central lesson of this chapter.

Pay attention to symptoms.

Pay attention to patterns.

And pay attention to what may happen before symptoms worsen.

That awareness may matter greatly.

Action Plan

- Think about whether you have noticed situations in which symptoms seem worse.

- Pay attention to repeated patterns.
- Write down possible triggers you have observed.
- Do not assume one trigger explains everything.
- Carry forward one important idea: recognizing triggers often begins by paying attention.

Transition to Chapter 7

Once you begin recognizing possible triggers, the next question becomes practical:

What can you do about them?

That is where we turn next.

CHAPTER 7: Reducing Triggers: Practical Prevention Strategies

Recognizing triggers is important.

But recognition alone is not enough.

The next question is practical:

What can you do about them?

That is where asthma management begins to move from understanding to action.

Because in many cases, better asthma control is not only about medicines.

It may also involve reducing exposures that aggravate symptoms.

And sometimes in ways patients underestimate.

The Goal Is Not to Control Everything

I want to begin with something important.

The goal is not perfection.

And it is not trying to control every detail of life.

That would be unrealistic.

And exhausting.

The goal is thoughtful risk reduction.

That is different.

And much more reasonable.

Good prevention is often about practical steps.

Not extreme measures.

Start With Triggers That Clearly Matter

Do not try to change everything at once.

Start with triggers that seem clearly relevant.

Especially repeated, recognizable triggers.

That is usually much smarter.

And much more sustainable.

Target what appears to matter.

That is often where the greatest benefit begins.

Reduce Exposure Where You Reasonably Can

This is the broad principle.

Reduce exposure where reasonable.

Not obsessively.

Reasonably.

That distinction matters.

Because reasonable prevention is often effective.

And much easier to live with.

Home Environment May Matter

Sometimes patients overlook this.

But everyday surroundings may matter.

And sometimes improvement begins with paying closer attention to ordinary environments.

That possibility deserves consideration.

Not alarm.

Consideration.

Workplace Exposures May Matter Too

Sometimes patterns at work may be important.

And if symptoms seem worse in certain environments, that deserves attention.

Patients sometimes recognize these patterns before anyone else.

Pay attention to what you notice.

That may matter.

Reducing Infection Risk May Be Part of Prevention

Because if respiratory infections seem to worsen asthma, prevention deserves thought.

That is a reasonable principle.

And often a practical one.

Because common problems deserve common-sense thinking.

Exercise Does Not Belong on an Avoidance List

I want to be very clear about this.

Reducing triggers is not the same as abandoning healthy activity.

Please do not conclude:

If exercise causes symptoms, I should avoid exercise.

That may be the wrong conclusion.

We will discuss exercise more fully later.

But for now, I want to make one point clear:

Reducing triggers is not the same as shrinking life.

Seasonal and Environmental Patterns May Call for Planning

Sometimes symptoms seem to follow predictable patterns.

If so, planning may help.

That is a practical point.

And a useful one.

Planning is often one of the most underrated tools in chronic illness.

Do not underestimate it.

Prevention Should Be Practical and Sustainable

This may be the heart of the chapter.

Practical.

Sustainable.

Not exhausting.

Not extreme.

Because strategies patients cannot live with are rarely good long-term strategies.

And long-term thinking matters.

Avoid Fear-Based Living

Sometimes patients become so focused on avoiding triggers that life starts shrinking.

That concerns me.

Because prevention should support living well.

Not undermine it.

Never let trigger awareness quietly turn into fear-based living.

That is too high a price.

And unnecessary.

Prevention Is Often About Reducing Risk, Not Eliminating Risk

Patients sometimes think prevention means eliminating all risk.

That is rarely realistic.

Often the goal is reducing risk.

And that is often achievable.

That is a much wiser framework.

And a much less burdensome one.

Why This Chapter Matters

Recognizing triggers without reducing them is incomplete.

And reducing relevant exposures may improve asthma control.

Sometimes substantially.

That is practical.

That is actionable.

Doctor's Pearl

Good trigger prevention is rarely about perfection.

It is usually about thoughtful, sustainable reduction of exposures that seem to matter.

Myth vs Fact

Myth: Preventing trigger exposure means avoiding large parts of normal life.

Fact: Good prevention is often about practical, reasonable steps, not extreme restriction.

Common Mistakes to Avoid

Trying to change everything at once.

Taking extreme measures that are not sustainable.

Confusing prevention with fear.

Assuming reducing triggers means abandoning healthy activities.

Ignoring patterns in home or work environments.

Red Flag Warnings

Discuss prevention strategies more carefully if:

- Symptoms keep worsening despite treatment
- Home or workplace exposures may be contributing
- Infections repeatedly seem linked to worsening
- Trigger avoidance has become driven by fear
- You feel unsure how to reduce exposures practically

These are important reasons to revisit prevention strategies.

Key Points

- Reducing triggers is a practical part of asthma management.
- The goal is reasonable risk reduction, not perfection.
- Start with triggers that clearly seem relevant.
- Prevention should be practical and sustainable.
- Planning often helps.
- Prevention should support living well, not shrink life.

Chapter Summary

Recognizing triggers matters.

But reducing relevant exposures matters too.

That is the central lesson of this chapter.

Good prevention is usually not about extreme restriction.

It is about thoughtful, practical steps that reduce risk and support better control.

And often, that can make a meaningful difference.

Action Plan

- Identify one or two triggers that seem most relevant to you.
- Focus first on practical steps, not drastic changes.
- Think about whether home, work, or seasonal patterns deserve attention.
- Avoid letting prevention turn into fear-based living.
- Carry forward one important idea: good prevention is practical, not perfect.

Transition to Chapter 8

Reducing triggers is one important part of asthma management.

But medicines may also play a major role.

How do asthma medicines work?

And why are there different kinds?

That is where we turn next.

CHAPTER 8: Asthma Medicines: Understanding Treatment

For many patients, this is where asthma begins to feel more real.

Medicines.

Inhalers.

Treatment decisions.

Questions.

Concerns.

Sometimes confusion.

And often understandable confusion.

Because asthma treatment may seem complicated at first.

Different medicines.

Different inhalers.

Different purposes.

Why so many?

Why not just one medicine for everything?

These are good questions.

And patients deserve clear answers.

Because treatment makes much more sense when you understand what asthma medicines are trying to do.

And why different medicines may serve different roles.

Asthma Treatment Often Has More Than One Goal

Patients sometimes think treatment has one purpose:

Relieve symptoms.

That is part of it.

But often not all of it.

Treatment may aim to:

- Relieve symptoms
- Help maintain control
- Reduce worsening or flare-ups
- Support better long-term stability

That broader view matters.

Because treatment is often about more than responding in the moment.

Sometimes it is about preventing problems too.

Not All Asthma Medicines Do the Same Thing

This is one of the most important ideas in this chapter.

Different medicines may serve different purposes.

Because confusion often begins when all medicines are assumed to do the same thing.

They do not.

And understanding that may reduce misunderstanding.

And sometimes improve treatment use.

Quick-Relief Medicines

Some medicines may be used to provide symptom relief.

Patients often understand these more easily.

Because the purpose feels obvious.

Symptoms.

Relief.

Immediate help.

That concept makes sense intuitively.

But it is only part of the larger treatment picture.

Medications for Asthma

Quick-Relief Medications

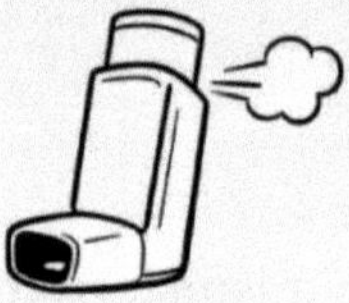

Quick-Relief Inhalers

- Albuterol
- Levalbuterol

Long-Term Control Medications

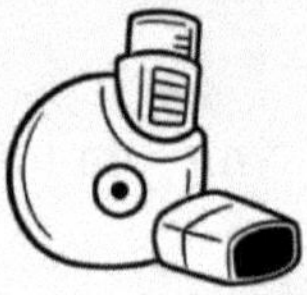

Combination Inhalers

- Fluticasone/Salmeterol
- Budesonide/Formoterol
- Fluticasone/Vilanterol

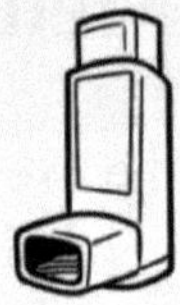

Inhaled Corticosteroids

- Fluticasone
- Budesonide
- Beclomethasone

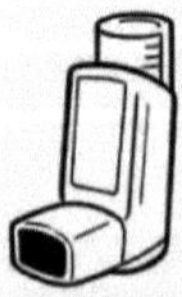

Inhaled Corticosteroids

- Fluticasone
- Budesonide
- Beclomethasone

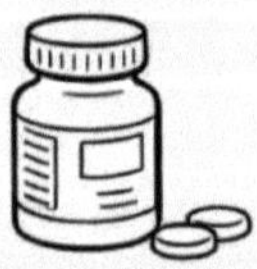

Oral Medications

- Montelukast
- Theophylline

Longer-Term Control Medicines

This is where confusion often begins.

Because some patients ask:

Why take treatment when I feel fine?

That is an important question.

Because some treatment approaches may relate not only to symptoms in the moment, but to maintaining control over time.

That is a different idea.

And an important one.

Why Treatment Plans May Differ

Patients sometimes compare treatments.

One person takes one medicine.

Another takes something different.

Why?

Because asthma may differ.

Severity may differ.

Needs may differ.

And treatment may therefore differ.

That is individualized medicine.

And often good medicine.

More Medicine Is Not Always Better Medicine

Patients sometimes assume stronger care means more medicines.

Be careful.

More is not automatically better.

Better is better.

Appropriate is better.

Thoughtful treatment is better.

That distinction matters.

Questions About Side Effects

Patients often worry about side effects.

And they should feel comfortable raising those concerns.

Always.

Questions about medicines should never be silenced by embarrassment or hesitation.

Questions improve care.

And that applies here too.

Do Not Make Independent Treatment Changes Casually

This is very important.

Please do not make major treatment decisions on your own based on fear.

Or assumptions.

Or internet confusion.

That can be risky.

Questions should lead to discussion.

Not impulsive decisions.

If Treatment Seems Confusing, Ask

If you do not understand why you are taking a medicine, ask.

If you do not understand the role of a medicine, ask.

If something does not make sense, ask.

Patients should understand treatment.

And good care should support that.

Treatment Is Often Part of a Bigger Strategy

Medicines matter.

But asthma management is often broader than medicines alone.

Triggers matter.

Monitoring matters.

Technique matters.

Preparedness matters.

That bigger picture matters.

And treatment makes more sense when seen within that larger framework.

Why This Chapter Matters

Treatment decisions affect daily life.

And patients should understand treatment.

Not simply receive it.

Understanding treatment often improves confidence.

And sometimes improves outcomes.

Doctor's Pearl

One of the most important things a patient can understand is this:

Not all asthma medicines serve the same purpose.

Understanding the role of treatment is part of good treatment.

Myth vs Fact

Myth: All asthma medicines basically do the same thing.

Fact: Different asthma medicines may serve different roles, and that distinction matters.

Common Mistakes to Avoid

Assuming all medicines have the same purpose.

Assuming feeling well means treatment questions no longer matter.

Changing treatment casually without discussion.

Staying silent when treatment does not make sense to you.

Assuming more medicine automatically means better care.

Red Flag Warnings

Discuss treatment questions promptly if:

- You do not understand why you are taking a medicine
- Treatment does not seem to be helping
- You have concerns about side effects

- You are considering changing treatment on your own
- Something about the treatment plan feels unclear

These are important reasons to reopen discussion.

Key Points

- Asthma treatment often has more than one goal.
- Different medicines may serve different purposes.
- Quick-relief and longer-term treatment approaches may play different roles.
- Treatment plans may differ because asthma differs.
- Questions about medicines matter.
- Patients should understand treatment, not simply receive it.

Chapter Summary

Asthma treatment may seem complicated at first.

But some of that complexity becomes clearer when you understand one central idea:

Different medicines may serve different purposes.

And treatment is often part of a broader strategy aimed not only at relieving symptoms, but supporting better control.

Understanding that is part of good asthma care.

Action Plan

- Review whether you understand the purpose of each asthma medicine you use.

- Write down any questions you have about treatment.
- If something about your treatment does not make sense, ask.
- Do not make independent treatment changes casually.
- Carry forward one important idea: understanding treatment is part of treatment.

Transition to Chapter 9

Understanding asthma medicines is important.

But another question is just as important:

Are inhalers being used correctly?

Because technique matters.

That is where we turn next.

CHAPTER 9: Using Inhalers Correctly: Why Technique Matters

This may be one of the most underestimated chapters in this book.

And yet, it may be one of the most important.

Because even good medicine may not help as intended if it is not used properly.

That is a simple idea.

But a powerful one.

Technique matters.

Sometimes more than people realize.

Because good treatment is not only about having the right medicine.

It may also depend on using that medicine well.

That distinction matters.

Good Medicine Still Depends on Good Use

Patients sometimes assume:

If I have the right inhaler, I am covered.

Maybe.

But not necessarily.

Because having the right medicine and using it effectively are not always the same thing.

And patients should understand that.

Because misunderstandings here may affect outcomes.

Sometimes substantially.

Technique Problems Are Not Uncommon

If inhaler technique needs improvement, that should not be a source of embarrassment.

Not at all.

Technique problems are not a personal failure.

They may be common.

And they may be fixable.

That is the important point.

Fixable.

And often easily improved.

That should be encouraging.

Small Technique Errors May Matter

This surprises some patients.

But small errors may matter.

Because inhaled treatment depends not only on the medicine itself, but on how it is delivered.

And delivery matters.

That is why technique deserves attention.

Even when things seem straightforward.

Do Not Assume You Are Using an Inhaler Correctly Simply Because You Have Used It for Years

I feel strongly about this.

Because I have seen patients use inhalers for years and still benefit from reviewing technique.

Please do not assume experience automatically means technique is perfect.

Be open to review.

That openness may help.

Sometimes significantly.

Ask to Have Technique Reviewed

This may be one of the most practical suggestions in the book.

Ask.

Have technique reviewed.

Have someone watch.

Have questions answered.

That is smart medicine.

And patients should feel entirely comfortable doing it.

If Treatment Seems Not to Be Working, Consider Technique

When treatment seems disappointing, people may assume:

The medicine failed.

Maybe.

But maybe technique deserves attention too.

That possibility should not be overlooked.

Because sometimes important answers hide in practical details.

How to Use an Inhaler

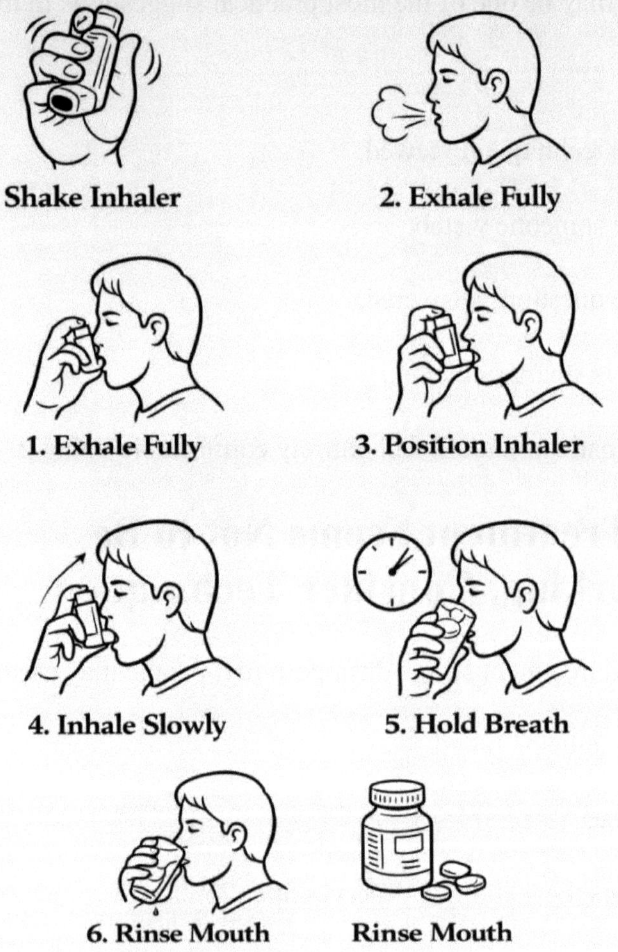

Inhaler Technique and Asthma Control May Be Connected

Technique may influence how well treatment works.

And how well asthma is controlled.

That possibility matters.

And it deserves respect.

Confidence Should Include Knowing How to Use Treatment Well

Confidence is not only about having medicines.

It is also about knowing how to use treatment properly.

That kind of confidence is stronger.

And more useful.

And patients deserve that.

Do Not Let Embarrassment Prevent Questions

Some patients hesitate to ask about inhaler use because they feel they should already know.

Please do not let pride interfere with good care.

Questions improve care.

Always.

And this is a perfect example.

Why Technique Matters Even More Than Patients Often Realize

Technique may influence whether treatment reaches its intended effect.

And if that matters, technique matters.

Sometimes profoundly.

That is why this chapter belongs in this book.

Why This Chapter Matters

Because inhaler technique may affect whether treatment works as intended.

Because technique problems may be common and fixable.

And because sometimes improving technique may improve outcomes.

That is practical.

That is actionable.

Doctor's Pearl

Never assume inhaler technique is too basic to revisit.

Sometimes reviewing basics leads to important improvements.

Myth vs Fact

Myth: If I have been using an inhaler for years, my technique must be correct.

Fact: Technique may be worth reviewing, even after years of use.

Common Mistakes to Avoid

Assuming having the right medicine automatically means it is being used effectively.

Assuming long experience guarantees correct technique.

Ignoring technique when treatment seems disappointing.

Feeling embarrassed to ask for technique review.

Treating inhaler use as too basic to matter.

Red Flag Warnings

Discuss technique review if:

- Treatment does not seem to be helping as expected
- Asthma control seems disappointing despite treatment
- You have never had inhaler technique reviewed
- You feel uncertain whether you are using the inhaler correctly
- You have questions about how your inhaler should be used

These are excellent reasons to revisit technique.

Key Points

- Good treatment still depends on good use.
- Inhaler technique problems may be common and fixable.
- Small technique errors may matter.
- Technique should be reviewed, not assumed.
- Technique may influence asthma control.
- Asking for technique review is smart medicine.

Chapter Summary

Using the right medicine matters.

But using it correctly may matter just as much.

That is the central lesson of this chapter.

Inhaler technique is not a minor detail.

It may influence whether treatment works as intended.

And because technique problems may be fixable, reviewing technique may sometimes lead to meaningful improvement.

That is worth remembering.

Action Plan

- Ask yourself whether your inhaler technique has ever been reviewed.
- If not, consider asking for a review.

- If treatment seems less effective than expected, consider whether technique deserves attention.
- Do not let embarrassment prevent questions.
- Carry forward one important idea: technique is part of treatment.

Transition to Chapter 10

Once treatment is in place, another question becomes very important:

How do you know whether your asthma is truly well controlled?

That is where we turn next.

CHAPTER 10: Is Your Asthma Well Controlled? Monitoring and Warning Signs

One of the most important questions in asthma care is often not asked often enough:

Is your asthma actually well controlled?

Not:

Are you surviving?

Not:

Are you simply getting by?

But:

Is your asthma well controlled?

That is a different question.

And an important one.

Because many people quietly accept more symptoms than they should.

And sometimes do not realize better control may be possible.

Because monitoring asthma is not about becoming preoccupied with illness.

It is about understanding how asthma is doing.

And recognizing when something may need attention.

That is thoughtful care.

What Does “Well Controlled” Mean?

Patients hear this phrase often.

But what does it actually mean?

In simple terms, good control generally means asthma is not intruding into life more than it should.

That is the broad idea.

Good control often means stability.

Predictability.

Confidence.

And fewer disruptions.

Symptoms May Be Telling You Something

Symptoms are not merely inconveniences.

Sometimes they are signals.

Signals worth noticing.

Because monitoring often begins by paying attention.

Thoughtfully.

Not anxiously.

Thoughtfully.

There is a difference.

Do Not Normalize Frequent Symptoms

I feel strongly about this.

Because patients sometimes quietly adapt to symptoms.

And begin assuming:

This is just how my asthma is.

Be careful.

That assumption may be wrong.

Frequent symptoms should not automatically be accepted as normal.

That deserves reflection.

And perhaps discussion.

Nighttime Symptoms Matter

Symptoms that disturb sleep deserve respect.

They may be telling you something important.

And should not be dismissed casually.

Never underestimate what nighttime symptoms may be trying to tell you.

Activity Limitation Matters

If asthma is quietly limiting what you do, that matters.

Even if you have adapted to it.

Especially if you have adapted to it.

Because adaptation sometimes hides problems.

And hidden problems deserve recognition.

Flare-Ups Are Part of the Monitoring Story

Monitoring is not only about day-to-day symptoms.

It also includes the bigger picture.

Patterns over time.

Instability.

Flare-ups.

These matter.

Because repeated worsening may be telling you something important.

Warning Signs Deserve Attention

Changes matter.

Worsening matters.

Patterns changing matters.

Patients should pay attention when asthma seems to be behaving differently.

That may be important.

Sometimes very important.

Monitoring Is Not Fear

I want to emphasize this.

Because I do not want patients confusing monitoring with living in worry.

They are not the same.

Monitoring is awareness.

Fear is something different.

Good monitoring supports confidence.

It should not undermine confidence.

Reassessment Is Part of Good Monitoring

Monitoring is not simply noticing symptoms.

It is also asking:

Does something need to be revisited?

That is wise.

Because good asthma care often includes reassessment.

And patients should understand that.

If You Are Unsure Whether Asthma Is Well Controlled, Ask

Ask.

Do not guess.

Do not assume.

Ask.

Questions about control are good questions.

And patients should feel comfortable raising them.

Always.

Why This Chapter Matters

Because monitoring helps patients recognize whether asthma is stable.

Or whether something may need attention.

Because recognizing change early may matter.

And because better control may sometimes be possible.

Doctor’s Pearl

One of the most important mistakes patients make is accepting symptoms as “normal” when better control may be possible.

Do not make that assumption too easily.

Myth vs Fact

Myth: If I am managing day to day, my asthma must be well controlled.

Fact: Getting by is not always the same as good control.

Common Mistakes to Avoid

Normalizing frequent symptoms.

Ignoring nighttime symptoms.

Overlooking activity limitation.

Confusing monitoring with fear.

Assuming better control is not possible.

Red Flag Warnings

Discuss reassessment promptly if:

- Symptoms are becoming more frequent
- Nighttime symptoms are occurring
- Asthma is limiting activity
- Flare-ups are recurring
- Asthma seems to be changing or worsening

These are important signals.

Pay attention to them.

Key Points

- Good asthma control means more than simply getting by.
- Symptoms may provide important signals.
- Frequent symptoms should not automatically be accepted as normal.
- Nighttime symptoms and activity limitation matter.
- Monitoring is about awareness, not fear.
- Reassessment is part of good asthma care.

Chapter Summary

Monitoring asthma is not about becoming preoccupied with illness.

It is about understanding how asthma is doing.

And recognizing when something may need attention.

That is the central lesson of this chapter.

Do not assume getting by means asthma is well controlled.

Better control may sometimes be possible.

And that matters.

Action Plan

- Reflect honestly on whether asthma may be intruding into life more than it should.
- Pay attention to symptoms, nighttime problems, and activity limitation.
- Do not normalize frequent symptoms too easily.
- If you are uncertain whether asthma is well controlled, ask.
- Carry forward one important idea: monitoring is part of good asthma care.

Transition to Chapter 11

If monitoring helps recognize when asthma is worsening, the next question becomes crucial:

What should you know about flare-ups and emergencies?

That is where we turn next.

CHAPTER 11: Asthma Flare-Ups and Emergencies: What You Should Know

Even when asthma is generally well managed, flare-ups may happen.

That is reality.

And patients should understand it.

Because good asthma care is not only about trying to prevent worsening.

It is also about knowing what to recognize if worsening occurs.

Preparation matters.

Recognition matters.

And understanding when asthma may be becoming more serious matters.

Sometimes urgently.

What Is a Flare-Up?

Patients use many words.

Attack.

Episode.

Bad asthma day.

Sudden worsening.

Flare-up.

The language varies.

But the general idea is worsening symptoms.

And patients should understand that concept.

Because recognizing worsening is often the first step in responding wisely.

Flare-Ups May Not Always Appear Dramatically at First

Patients sometimes imagine emergencies always arrive suddenly and obviously.

Sometimes they do.

Sometimes they may not.

Sometimes worsening may develop progressively.

And that possibility matters.

Because subtle worsening may still deserve attention.

Never assume only dramatic symptoms matter.

Pay Attention When Asthma Is Behaving Differently

Change matters.

If asthma seems different.

Worse.

Less predictable.

Harder to settle.

Pay attention.

That may be important.

Patients often recognize change before they fully understand what it means.

Trust that observation enough to take it seriously.

Do Not Minimize Worsening Symptoms

This is a mistake I worry about.

People sometimes explain worsening away.

Wait too long.

Hope it will simply pass.

Please be careful.

Minimizing worsening may be risky.

Especially when symptoms seem to be progressing.

Repeated Flare-Ups Matter

Even if symptoms improve, repeated worsening deserves attention.

Because repeated flare-ups may be telling you something.

Perhaps monitoring needs review.

Perhaps triggers need reassessment.

Perhaps treatment deserves rethinking.

Repeated worsening should not be dismissed casually.

Emergencies Deserve Respect

I want to say this plainly.

Serious breathing distress is serious.

Do not underestimate it.

Do not delay when urgent help may be needed.

This is not the place for hesitation driven by pride.

Or denial.

Or wishful thinking.

Be careful.

Preparedness Matters Before a Problem Happens

Preparedness works best before it is needed.

Not in the middle of panic.

Before.

That matters.

Because clarity is often harder during distress.

Preparation beforehand may help.

Sometimes greatly.

An Asthma Action Plan May Be Very Valuable

Structured planning may help some patients.

And planning often reduces confusion.

Especially when symptoms worsen.

Patients should at least know this concept exists.

Because it may be valuable.

Asthma Flare-Ups

Here's what to do if your asthma gets worse suddenly.

1. Stay Calm and Sit Up

Try to stay calm, sit upright, and take deep breaths.

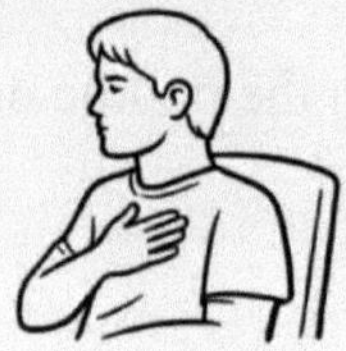

2. Use Your Quick-Relief Inhaler

Take 1-2 puffs of your quick-relief inhaler, like albuterol. Follow your asthma action plan for specific instructions.

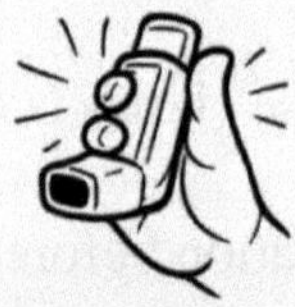

3. Recheck Symptoms

Wait a few minutes and see if your symptoms improve. You may take more puffs if needed, as directed by your asthma action plan.

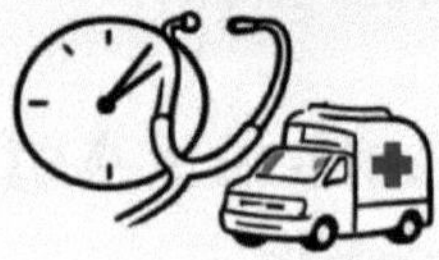

4. Seek Medical Help If Needed

If symptoms get worse or don't get better, get medical help right away.
Call your doctor or go to the emergency room.

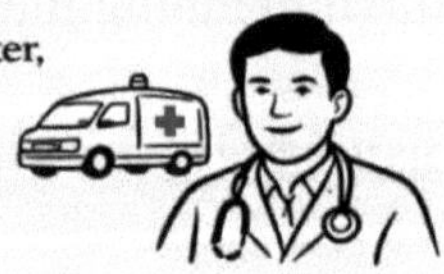

Do Not Let Fear Prevent Good Decisions

Emergencies can trigger hesitation.

Or denial.

Or delay.

Do not let fear quietly interfere with wise action.

That is a very important principle.

If You Are Unsure Whether a Situation Is Serious, Take That Seriously

If you are seriously unsure whether symptoms may be becoming dangerous, do not dismiss that uncertainty.

Take it seriously.

That instinct may matter.

Sometimes enormously.

Why This Chapter Matters

Because worsening symptoms may happen.

Because recognition matters.

Because preparedness matters.

And because emergencies deserve respect.

Doctor's Pearl

One of the most dangerous assumptions in asthma is:

I will wait a little longer.

Be very careful with delay when symptoms may be worsening seriously.

Myth vs Fact

Myth: Asthma emergencies always appear suddenly and unmistakably.

Fact: Sometimes worsening may develop progressively, and recognizing change early may matter greatly.

Common Mistakes to Avoid

Minimizing worsening symptoms.

Waiting too long.

Assuming repeated flare-ups do not matter.

Ignoring the value of preparedness.

Letting uncertainty lead to delay.

Red Flag Warnings

Seek urgent medical attention if:

- Breathing distress feels severe or rapidly worsening
- Symptoms feel frighteningly different from usual
- Breathing difficulty is interfering with speaking or functioning
- Usual measures do not seem to be helping
- You are seriously concerned you may be dealing with an emergency

Do not ignore severe breathing distress.

Key Points

- Flare-ups may happen even when asthma is generally well managed.
- Worsening may not always begin dramatically.
- Change in symptom patterns matters.
- Repeated flare-ups deserve attention.
- Preparedness matters.
- Emergencies deserve respect.
- Delay may be dangerous.

Chapter Summary

Asthma flare-ups may happen.

And patients should be prepared for that possibility.

That is the central lesson of this chapter.

Recognize worsening.

Respect change.

Take repeated flare-ups seriously.

And do not delay when serious symptoms may need urgent attention.

Preparedness matters.

And sometimes it may matter enormously.

Action Plan

- Think about whether you know how you would respond if asthma worsened significantly.
- Ask whether an asthma action plan would be helpful.
- Take repeated flare-ups seriously.
- Do not minimize serious worsening.
- Carry forward one important idea: preparedness is part of good asthma care.

Transition to Chapter 12

Asthma is not only about symptoms and emergencies.

It is also about living.

Working.

Exercising.

Traveling.

Living fully.

That is where we turn next.

CHAPTER 12: Living an Active Life With Asthma

One of the quiet fears many patients carry is this:

Will asthma make my life smaller?

It is a deeply human question.

And an important one.

Because chronic illness does not raise only medical questions.

It raises life questions.

Can I exercise?

Can I travel?

Can I work normally?

Can I live fully?

Patients deserve honest discussion about those questions.

Because asthma care is not only about reducing symptoms.

It is also about preserving life as fully as possible.

Do Not Assume Asthma Means Automatic Limitation

Please do not assume asthma automatically means major restriction.

Be very careful with that assumption.

It may be wrong.

And unnecessarily discouraging.

Because fear sometimes limits life more than asthma itself.

And that deserves recognition.

Activity Matters

Some patients begin pulling back from life too early.

Doing less.

Trying less.

Trusting their bodies less.

That concerns me.

Because unnecessary retreat can become its own burden.

And patients should be careful about that.

Exercise and Asthma

Patients often worry about exercise.

Understandably.

But exercise should not automatically be viewed as the enemy.

Please do not think that way.

Exercise may raise practical questions.

But questions should lead to thoughtful management.

Not automatic avoidance.

That distinction matters greatly.

Work and Daily Life

Asthma may raise practical questions about work and daily routines.

That is real.

But practical questions do not automatically mean impossible obstacles.

Please do not assume they do.

Sometimes thoughtful planning matters.

Sometimes practical adjustments matter.

That is different from surrender.

Very different.

Travel and Asthma

Patients ask about travel often.

And I understand why.

Travel can raise uncertainty.

But I do not want patients assuming asthma automatically closes that door.

Planning often changes what feels possible.

And patients should not underestimate the power of planning.

Confidence Matters

Confidence matters.

Not false confidence.

Real confidence.

Confidence built through understanding.

Preparedness.

Experience.

Thoughtful care.

That kind of confidence matters.

And may help restore freedom that fear has quietly narrowed.

Do Not Let Fear Quietly Take Over

Fear can be subtle.

Sometimes it simply persuades people to do less.

Risk less.

Live smaller.

Be alert to that.

Because that may happen quietly.

And it deserves resistance.

Thoughtful resistance.

Living Actively Does Not Mean Ignoring Asthma

This is important balance.

I am not suggesting denial.

Or recklessness.

Living actively does not mean pretending asthma does not exist.

It means not letting asthma define the limits of life unnecessarily.

That is very different.

Sometimes the Right Question Is Not "Can I?"

But "How Can I?"

This changes perspective.

Sometimes patients ask:

Can I exercise?

Can I travel?

Can I do this?

Sometimes the better question is:

How can I do it wisely?

That is often a much more constructive question.

And often a much more hopeful one.

Living Well Is Part of Asthma Care

Sometimes chronic disease discussions become too narrow.

Too focused on symptoms alone.

Too little focused on life.

That is incomplete.

Living well is part of asthma care.

It should be seen that way.

Why This Chapter Matters

Because asthma should not be discussed only in terms of limitations.

That is too narrow.

Patients deserve discussion about possibility too.

And that is what this chapter is about.

Possibility.

Thoughtful possibility.

Doctor's Pearl

One of the most harmful assumptions a patient can make is:

Asthma means I should quietly do less.

Be very careful with that assumption.

It may be profoundly wrong.

Myth vs Fact

Myth: If I have asthma, I should probably avoid an active life.

Fact: In many cases, thoughtful management may help support an active, full life.

Common Mistakes to Avoid

Assuming asthma automatically means major limitation.

Letting fear quietly narrow life.

Confusing thoughtful caution with unnecessary retreat.

Assuming questions about activity mean activity is impossible.

Forgetting that planning often changes what feels possible.

Red Flag Warnings

Discuss reassessment if:

- Asthma is limiting activity more than it should
- Fear is causing you to withdraw from important parts of life
- Exercise or daily activities raise unresolved concerns
- You have quietly accepted limitations you have never questioned

These are important reasons to reopen discussion.

Key Points

- Asthma does not automatically mean major limitation.
- Activity matters.
- Exercise should not automatically be viewed as the enemy.
- Planning may help preserve work, travel, and daily life.
- Confidence matters.
- Fear should not quietly define the limits of life.
- Living well is part of asthma care.

Chapter Summary

Asthma may raise practical questions about exercise, work, travel, and daily living.

But those questions should not automatically be answered with limitation.

That is the central lesson of this chapter.

Be careful what assumptions you accept.

Because thoughtful management, planning, and confidence may preserve far more possibility than fear sometimes suggests.

Action Plan

- Reflect honestly on whether fear may have narrowed any part of your life.
- Revisit any limitations you may have quietly accepted.
- Ask not only "Can I?" but also "How can I do this wisely?"
- Think about whether planning could restore possibilities you may have assumed were lost.
- Carry forward one important idea: living well is part of asthma care.

Transition to Chapter 13

Sometimes asthma is not the whole story.

Sometimes other conditions may affect symptoms or control.

That is where we turn next.

CHAPTER 13: When Asthma Is Not the Whole Story

Sometimes asthma is the diagnosis.

But not the whole story.

And patients should understand that.

Because sometimes asthma may coexist with other conditions.

And those other conditions may matter.

Sometimes greatly.

Because when asthma seems harder to control than expected, it may be wise to ask:

Is something else also contributing?

That is a smart question.

Sometimes More Than One Thing May Be Going On

Medicine is not always simple.

Not always one diagnosis.

One explanation.

One problem.

Sometimes more than one thing may be present.

And patients should understand that possibility.

Because it may help explain why symptoms sometimes seem more complicated than expected.

When Asthma Seems Harder to Control Than It Should

If asthma seems unusually difficult to control.

If symptoms keep recurring.

If progress seems disappointing.

It may be reasonable to ask whether something else deserves consideration.

That is not pessimism.

That is thoughtful medicine.

Allergies May Sometimes Affect the Picture

We have discussed allergies before.

They matter here too.

Because sometimes overlapping issues may influence symptoms or control.

And when overlap exists, recognizing it may matter.

Acid Reflux May Sometimes Matter

Patients are sometimes surprised by this.

But they should at least know the question exists.

Because sometimes overlapping issues deserve consideration.

And when something overlaps, understanding that may matter.

Upper Airway or Nasal Issues May Sometimes Matter

Sometimes the breathing story is broader than patients realize.

And broader thinking may matter.

That is the point of this chapter.

Broad thinking.

Not narrow assumptions.

Sleep-Related Issues May Sometimes Matter

This may be relevant in some patients.

And patients should at least know that possibility exists.

Because sometimes symptoms that seem straightforward may deserve deeper thinking.

Anxiety, Stress, and Symptom Experience

This requires care.

And respect.

I do not want symptoms minimized.

Ever.

But patients should understand that life factors may sometimes affect symptom experience.

And that thoughtful discussion of those possibilities is not dismissal.

It is thoughtful care.

Sometimes Overlap May Help Explain Persistent Symptoms

This may be one of the central ideas of this chapter.

Overlap may matter.

And sometimes recognizing overlap helps make sense of symptoms that otherwise seem puzzling.

That may be very important.

If Asthma Seems Hard to Control, Ask Broader Questions

Ask broader questions.

Could something else be contributing?

Could overlap matter?

Could something deserve reevaluation?

These are smart questions.

And sometimes very important questions.

This Is Not About Making Things Seem More Complicated

This chapter is not meant to make asthma feel overwhelming.

Quite the opposite.

It is meant to make difficult situations make more sense.

That is different.

And much more helpful.

Why This Chapter Matters

Sometimes asthma is not the whole story.

And if something else is contributing, recognizing that may matter greatly.

This chapter encourages broader thinking.

And broader thinking is often part of good medicine.

Doctor's Pearl

When asthma seems harder to control than expected, one of the smartest questions to ask is:

Could something else also be contributing?

Never underestimate that question.

Myth vs Fact

Myth: If asthma symptoms persist, the answer must simply be stronger asthma treatment.

Fact: Sometimes persistent symptoms may raise questions about overlapping conditions that deserve consideration.

Common Mistakes to Avoid

Assuming asthma is always the whole explanation.

Assuming persistent symptoms simply mean "more asthma."

Failing to ask broader questions when control seems disappointing.

Confusing broader evaluation with unnecessary complication.

Red Flag Warnings

Discuss broader evaluation if:

- Asthma seems unusually hard to control
- Symptoms keep recurring despite treatment
- Something about the picture seems confusing
- Progress seems disappointing despite serious effort
- You have never asked whether overlapping issues may matter

These are excellent reasons to look deeper.

Key Points

- Sometimes asthma may not be the whole story.
- More than one condition may sometimes be contributing.
- Overlapping issues may affect symptoms or control.
- Persistent symptoms may sometimes call for broader thinking.
- Asking broader questions may be wise.
- Broader evaluation is often part of good medicine.

Chapter Summary

Sometimes asthma is not the whole story.

That is the central lesson of this chapter.

When symptoms seem harder to control than expected, it may be wise to ask whether something else may also be contributing.

That is not pessimism.

That is thoughtful medicine.

And sometimes it may matter greatly.

Action Plan

- If asthma has seemed harder to control than expected, ask whether broader questions deserve discussion.
- Reflect on whether symptoms have ever seemed more complicated than simple asthma alone.
- Do not assume persistent symptoms always mean "more asthma."
- Carry forward one important idea: broader thinking may sometimes lead to better answers.

Transition to Chapter 14

Sometimes broader evaluation raises another important question:

Could asthma be moving beyond routine management?

That is where we turn next.

CHAPTER 14: When Asthma Is Severe: Recognizing When Usual Approaches Are Not Enough

Most people with asthma can achieve good control.

That is important to say at the outset.

Because this chapter is not meant to alarm readers.

It is meant to inform them.

Thoughtfully.

Honestly.

And, I hope, reassuringly.

But it is also true that some patients may have asthma that is unusually difficult to control.

And patients should understand that possibility.

Because recognizing difficulty matters.

Difficult-to-Control Asthma Is Not Always the Same as Severe Asthma

This is very important.

Because these terms are often used loosely.

And they should not be.

Sometimes asthma seems difficult to control because something important has not yet been fully addressed.

Technique.

Triggers.

Adherence.

Overlapping conditions.

We have discussed these.

And they matter here.

Because sometimes asthma that seems severe may deserve deeper reassessment before such a conclusion is assumed.

When Asthma Seems Hard to Control, Ask Why

Do not assume persistent difficulty automatically means severe asthma.

Ask why.

Ask what deserves review.

Ask whether something important has been overlooked.

These are smart questions.

And sometimes they lead to important answers.

Repeated Flare-Ups Matter

Repeated worsening deserves attention.

Especially when it keeps happening.

Because repeated flare-ups may be telling you something.

Perhaps current management needs reassessment.

Perhaps deeper evaluation deserves discussion.

Repeated instability should not be dismissed casually.

If Asthma Is Limiting Life Significantly, Pay Attention

If asthma is seriously affecting sleep.

Activity.

Daily function.

Confidence.

Quality of life.

That deserves attention.

Because that burden should not be quietly accepted as inevitable.

Be careful about accepting too much as normal.

Specialist Evaluation May Matter

Some patients hesitate to seek specialist evaluation.

Please do not assume needing expertise means failure.

It does not.

Sometimes specialist evaluation is exactly the right next step.

And sometimes a very important one.

Expertise matters.

Especially when the picture is complicated.

Do Not Accept Poor Control Casually

Some patients gradually lower expectations.

Adapt to too many symptoms.

Accept too much instability.

Please be careful.

Poor control should not be accepted casually.

Especially when deeper evaluation may be warranted.

Severe Asthma Is Not a Personal Failure

This needs to be said clearly.

Difficulty controlling asthma is not a character failure.

Not a personal failure.

Not proof you have done something wrong.

Medicine should never be framed that way.

Ever.

What matters is recognizing difficulty.

And responding thoughtfully.

Recognition Matters Because It May Lead to Better Answers

Recognition matters.

Because recognizing a problem is often the first step toward addressing it wisely.

And patients should understand that.

Why This Chapter Matters

Some patients may need to recognize when asthma may be moving beyond routine management.

And recognizing that possibility may matter greatly.

This is a chapter about recognition.

And recognition matters.

Doctor's Pearl

If asthma remains difficult to control despite serious effort, do not simply assume this is something you must live with.

Ask whether deeper evaluation is needed.

That question may matter greatly.

Myth vs Fact

Myth: If asthma remains poorly controlled, there is probably little more to understand.

Fact: Persistent difficulty may be a reason to look deeper, not stop asking questions.

Common Mistakes to Avoid

Assuming difficult control automatically means severe asthma.

Accepting poor control as inevitable.

Ignoring repeated flare-ups.

Avoiding specialist evaluation when it may be appropriate.

Treating difficulty as personal failure.

Red Flag Warnings

Discuss deeper evaluation if:

- Asthma remains difficult to control despite serious effort
- Flare-ups keep recurring
- Asthma is significantly limiting daily life
- Symptoms seem increasingly unstable
- You suspect routine management may not be enough

These are important reasons to look deeper.

Key Points

- Difficult-to-control asthma and severe asthma are not always the same.
- Persistent difficulty should prompt deeper questions.
- Repeated flare-ups matter.
- Major impact on daily life deserves attention.
- Specialist evaluation may be important.
- Poor control should not be accepted casually.
- Recognition may be the first step toward better answers.

Chapter Summary

Most asthma can be managed well.

But some patients may have asthma that is unusually difficult to control.

And recognizing that possibility matters.

That is the central lesson of this chapter.

Do not assume persistent difficulty should simply be accepted.

Ask deeper questions.

Seek deeper evaluation.

Because recognition may be where better answers begin.

Action Plan

- If asthma seems unusually difficult to control, ask why.
- Make sure correctable issues have been reviewed.
- Take repeated flare-ups seriously.
- If poor control is significantly affecting life, raise that concern.
- Carry forward one important idea: recognizing difficult asthma may be the first step toward better answers.

Transition to Chapter 15

If asthma may be moving beyond routine management, the next question naturally follows:

What additional options may exist?

That is where we turn next.

CHAPTER 15: Newer and Advanced Treatments for Asthma: Progress, Possibilities, and Grounded Hope

One of the quiet fears some patients carry is this:

What if the usual treatments are not enough for me?

That is a real fear.

And a reasonable one.

But it deserves a thoughtful answer.

And the answer is this:

Asthma care has evolved.

Important advances have occurred.

And in some patients, newer and more advanced treatment approaches may matter.

Because difficulty does not automatically mean there are no options.

And patients should understand that.

Asthma Treatment Has Changed

Patients sometimes assume asthma care today is basically what it has always been.

It is not.

Understanding has grown.

Treatment has evolved.

Specialized care has advanced.

That is real progress.

And real progress deserves recognition.

Because it changes perspective.

This Chapter Is About Possibilities, Not Promises

I want to make that clear.

Because I do not want this chapter misunderstood.

This is not a chapter of exaggerated claims.

Or unrealistic promises.

It is a chapter about possibilities.

Thoughtful possibilities.

Grounded possibilities.

That is different.

And much more trustworthy.

Newer Treatment Approaches May Matter in Some Patients

In some situations, additional options may become relevant.

That possibility matters.

And it deserves awareness.

Because patients facing difficult asthma should not automatically assume the conversation has ended.

Sometimes it may be expanding.

Precision Medicine and Individualized Care

Patients may hear terms like precision medicine.

Do not let terminology obscure the simple idea.

The idea is individualized care.

Moving away from one-size-fits-all thinking.

And toward care better tailored to the individual.

That is the idea.

And it is an important one.

Progress Is Not Only About New Medicines

Patients sometimes think progress means only new drugs.

That is too narrow.

Progress may also involve:

- Better understanding
- Better personalization
- Better strategies
- Better systems of care

All of these may matter.

And patients should understand that.

Advanced Treatment Is Not a Sign of Failure

This needs to be said.

Clearly.

Because some patients quietly think:

If I need more advanced treatment, I must have failed somehow.

Please reject that idea.

It is wrong.

Medicine is not a moral test.

Using more advanced treatment when appropriate is not failure.

It is care.

Thoughtful care.

Hope Matters Here

This may be the heart of the chapter.

Hope matters.

Not hype.

Not false promises.

Grounded hope.

That is different.

And much better.

Because patients facing difficult asthma deserve honesty.

But they also deserve perspective.

And perspective may include hope.

Newer and Advanced Asthma Treatments

Here are some newer and advanced treatment options for asthma:

1. Biologic Therapies

Targeted injections like dupilumab, mepolizumab, benralizumab, which help control inflammation.

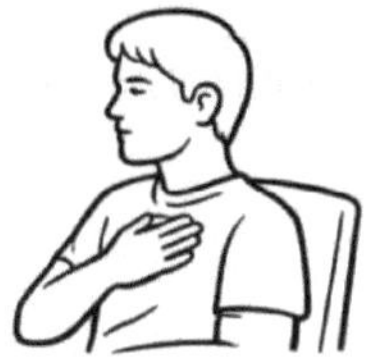

2. Bronchial Thermoplasty

A procedure using heat to reduce the smooth muscle in the airways, making them less likely to tighten.

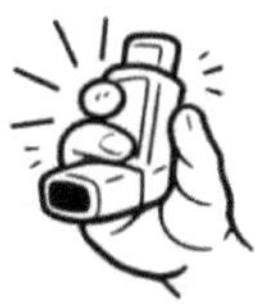

3. New Bronchodilators

Includes newer long-acting inhalers such as long-acting muscarinic antagonists (LAMAs) that help keep airways relaxed.

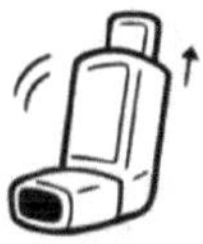

4. Smart Inhalers

Inhalers with sensors that track usage and symptoms through smartphone apps to help manage asthma better.

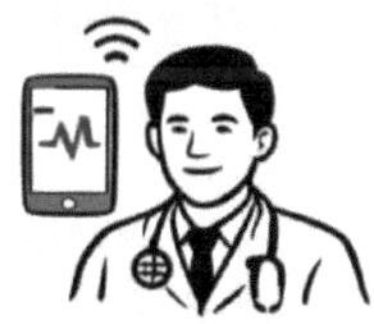

Do Not Assume Current Limits Define Future Possibilities

Do not assume that.

Ever.

Current difficulty does not automatically define the limits of what may be possible.

Be very careful with that assumption.

It may be wrong.

And unnecessarily discouraging.

Stay Engaged

Stay engaged.

Ask questions.

Stay curious.

Ask whether additional options deserve discussion.

That is wise.

And sometimes very important.

Patients who remain engaged often benefit most from progress.

Why This Chapter Matters

Patients should know asthma care continues to evolve.

Progress exists.

And for some patients, that progress may matter greatly.

This is a chapter about possibility.

And grounded hope.

Doctor's Pearl

Never assume current limitations define the limits of what may be possible.

Medicine has often proved that assumption wrong.

Myth vs Fact

Myth: If usual asthma treatment has not been enough, there is probably little else to consider.

Fact: Asthma care has advanced, and additional possibilities may sometimes exist.

Common Mistakes to Avoid

Assuming difficult asthma means no options remain.

Confusing advanced treatment with failure.

Confusing hope with hype.

Disengaging because current treatment feels disappointing.

Assuming progress means only new medicines.

Red Flag Warnings

Reopen discussion if:

- Asthma remains difficult despite serious effort
- You have never asked whether additional options deserve discussion
- Discouragement has led to resignation
- You assume current limitations define all future possibilities

These are important moments to ask deeper questions.

Key Points

- Asthma care has evolved.
- Newer and advanced approaches may matter in some patients.
- Progress is not only about new medicines.
- Advanced treatment is not failure.
- Grounded hope is different from hype.
- Current difficulty does not necessarily define future possibilities.
- Staying engaged matters.

Chapter Summary

Asthma care has advanced.

And that is the central message of this chapter.

For some patients, that progress may matter greatly.

The important lesson is simple:

Do not assume current difficulty means the end of options.

It may not.

And that possibility is worth understanding.

Action Plan

- If asthma has been difficult to control, ask whether additional options deserve discussion.
- Do not assume current limitations define future possibilities.
- Stay engaged and ask questions.
- Distinguish between grounded hope and exaggerated claims.
- Carry forward one important idea: progress may matter.

Transition to Chapter 16

Asthma may raise different questions at different stages of life.

Children.

Older adults.

Pregnancy.

These situations deserve special attention.

That is where we turn next.

CHAPTER 16: Asthma in Special Situations: Children, Older Adults, and Pregnancy

Asthma is a common condition.

But it does not always raise the same questions in every stage of life.

And it does not always look quite the same either.

That matters.

Because a parent worrying about a child with asthma may have different concerns than an older adult developing breathing symptoms later in life.

And pregnancy may raise its own important questions.

All of those concerns deserve thoughtful discussion.

Because good asthma care sometimes means recognizing when the usual conversation needs to be adapted to special situations.

Asthma in Children

Few things worry parents more than seeing a child struggle to breathe.

That is deeply understandable.

And it deserves acknowledgment.

But I want to begin with reassurance.

Many children with asthma can do very well.

Very well.

That matters to say clearly.

Because fear can easily outrun facts.

And parents deserve perspective.

Children Can Often Live Active Lives

Asthma in a child should not automatically mean a life of constant restriction.

Please do not assume that.

Children often can play.

Participate.

Be active.

And thrive.

That possibility matters enormously.

Parents Should Pay Attention to Patterns

As with adults, patterns matter.

Cough.

Wheezing.

Nighttime symptoms.

Exercise symptoms.

Repeated breathing problems.

These patterns may matter.

And parents often notice important patterns before anyone else.

That observational role matters.

Asthma in Older Adults

Asthma in older adults may raise somewhat different considerations.

Symptoms may be interpreted differently.

Other conditions may complicate the picture.

Diagnosis may sometimes require especially thoughtful evaluation.

That matters.

And should not be overlooked.

Do Not Assume New Breathing Symptoms Are "Just Age"

I feel strongly about this.

Because I have seen symptoms dismissed too casually.

Breathlessness should not be explained away carelessly.

If new breathing symptoms develop later in life, they deserve thoughtful evaluation.

That is simply good medicine.

More Than One Thing May Be Going On

This connects with earlier chapters.

And it matters here too.

Sometimes asthma may coexist with other conditions.

And that possibility may affect evaluation and care.

That deserves respect.

Because layered medicine is often real medicine.

Asthma and Pregnancy

This is an area where questions are common.

And understandable.

Patients may wonder:

What happens to asthma during pregnancy?

Will asthma affect pregnancy?

Are treatments safe?

These are important questions.

And they deserve individualized discussion.

Very individualized discussion.

Because pregnancy deserves thoughtful care.

Always.

Do Not Make Independent Treatment Decisions During Pregnancy

This is very important.

Please do not make major asthma treatment decisions during pregnancy based on fear.

Or assumptions.

Or internet confusion.

Discuss questions thoughtfully.

That is the safer approach.

And the wiser one.

Planning Matters in Special Situations

Planning matters.

Whether the patient is a child.

An older adult.

Or someone navigating pregnancy.

Preparedness helps.

Follow-up helps.

Thoughtful discussion helps.

These principles travel well.

Across every stage of life.

The Core Principles Still Remain the Same

Even in special situations, the fundamentals still matter.

Good diagnosis.

Good monitoring.

Good technique.

Good communication.

Good reassessment.

Those principles do not disappear.

They remain central.

That is reassuring.

Because it means the foundation still holds.

Why This Chapter Matters

Asthma may raise different questions in different stages of life.

And those questions deserve thoughtful attention.

Parents need reassurance.

Older adults need careful evaluation.

And pregnancy deserves individualized discussion.

Doctor's Pearl

Special situations may change the questions.

But they do not change the importance of thoughtful, individualized asthma care.

Myth vs Fact

Myth: Asthma in children, older adults, or pregnancy is too complicated for ordinary patients to understand.

Fact: The principles can be understood, and thoughtful discussion helps greatly.

Common Mistakes to Avoid

Assuming asthma in children automatically means major lifelong limitation.

Dismissing new breathing symptoms later in life as "just age."

Making independent treatment decisions during pregnancy based on fear.

Assuming the core principles of asthma care no longer apply in special situations.

Red Flag Warnings

Discuss reassessment if:

- A child has repeated breathing symptoms or recurrent concerns
- New breathing symptoms develop later in life
- Asthma seems harder to control during pregnancy
- You are uncertain how asthma care should be approached in a special situation
- Something about the picture feels unclear

These are important reasons to ask questions.

Key Points

- Asthma may raise different questions in children, older adults, and pregnancy.

- Many children with asthma can do very well.
- New breathing symptoms later in life deserve thoughtful evaluation.
- More than one condition may sometimes be present.
- Pregnancy-related asthma questions deserve individualized discussion.
- Planning and preparedness matter.
- The core principles of asthma care still apply.

Chapter Summary

Asthma may raise different concerns at different stages of life.

That is the central lesson of this chapter.

But the broader message is reassuring.

The principles of good asthma care remain.

Thoughtful evaluation.

Good communication.

Planning.

Reassessment.

These still matter.

And they still help.

Action Plan

- If asthma involves a child, pay attention to patterns and ask questions.

- If new breathing symptoms develop later in life, do not dismiss them casually.
- If pregnancy raises questions about asthma care, seek individualized discussion.
- Do not make important treatment decisions in special situations based on assumptions.
- Carry forward one important idea: the core principles of asthma care still apply.

Transition to Chapter 17

We have discussed diagnosis.

Triggers.

Treatment.

Monitoring.

Severe asthma.

And special situations.

Now we turn to a broader question:

What does the future of asthma care look like?

That is where we turn next.

CHAPTER 17: The Future of Asthma Care: New Science, New Possibilities, and Realistic Hope

When people live with a chronic illness, one question sometimes sits quietly in the background:

Will things get better?

That is a human question.

And a reasonable one.

This chapter is about that question.

And about answering it honestly.

Not with hype.

Not with false promises.

But with perspective.

And grounded hope.

Because hope matters.

Especially when it is rooted in reality.

Asthma Care Has Already Changed

Patients sometimes think of “the future” as something distant.

But in some ways, the future has already been arriving.

Understanding has improved.

Treatment has evolved.

Specialized care has advanced.

That is real progress.

And recognizing progress matters.

Because it reminds patients that medicine does not stand still.

Better Understanding Often Leads to Better Care

Sometimes the most important advances begin with deeper understanding.

And that has happened in asthma.

Understanding of inflammation.

Different asthma patterns.

Individualized care.

These advances matter.

Because better understanding often leads to better decisions.

And better decisions often lead to better outcomes.

That is often how progress happens.

Step by step.

Precision Medicine and Individualized Care

We touched on this earlier.

It belongs here too.

Because it may be part of the future.

Move beyond one-size-fits-all thinking.

And toward care better tailored to the individual.

That is the idea.

And it is an important one.

The Future Is Not Only About New Drugs

Patients sometimes think the future of medicine means only new medicines.

That is too narrow.

The future may also involve:

- Better diagnosis
- Better monitoring
- Better personalization
- Better prevention
- Better systems of care

All of these may matter.

And patients should understand that.

Technology May Play a Growing Role

Technology may influence:

- Monitoring
- Communication
- Self-management support
- Better use of information

The details may evolve.

But the broader idea is worth understanding.

The future may include not only better treatments.

But smarter care.

Research Continues

Work continues.

Questions continue.

Discovery continues.

Because it means the future is not idle.

It is being worked on.

Right now.

That is worth knowing.

Realistic Hope Is Better Than Hype

Medicine sometimes attracts exaggerated claims.

Be careful.

False promises help no one.

Realistic hope is better.

Much better.

Realistic hope says:

Progress is happening.

Understanding is growing.

Options may expand.

Care may improve.

That is meaningful.

And honest.

What This Means for Patients Today

Some readers may ask:

What does any of this mean for me now?

Fair question.

It means do not assume today's challenges define tomorrow's possibilities.

Do not assume asthma care is frozen.

Stay engaged.

Stay curious.

Ask questions.

Because patients who remain engaged often benefit most from progress.

The Future Is Also Better Partnership

Sometimes the future of care is not a distant breakthrough.

Sometimes it is better partnership.

Better communication.

Better follow-up.

Better decisions.

Sometimes the future begins there.

In ordinary good care.

That matters too.

Why This Chapter Matters

Chronic illness can sometimes narrow perspective.

And patients may quietly assume today is as good as it gets.

This chapter challenges that assumption.

Because progress exists.

And possibility exists.

And that is worth recognizing.

Doctor's Pearl

Never assume current limitations define the limits of what may be possible in the future.

Medicine has often proved that assumption wrong.

Myth vs Fact

Myth: Asthma treatment has basically reached its limits.

Fact: Asthma care continues to evolve, and important progress continues.

Common Mistakes to Avoid

Assuming nothing new is happening in asthma care.

Confusing hope with hype.

Disengaging because asthma feels “already figured out.”

Thinking the future only means new drugs.

Red Flag Warnings

Reopen discussion if:

- You feel current options have been exhausted
- You have difficult-to-control asthma
- You have never asked whether newer approaches may be relevant
- Discouragement has led to resignation

These may be exactly the moments when renewed discussion matters.

Key Points

- Asthma care has evolved.
- Better understanding has led to important progress.
- The future may involve better diagnosis, monitoring, personalization, prevention, and systems of care.
- Technology may play a growing role.
- Realistic hope is better than hype.
- Staying engaged may help patients benefit from progress.
- The future of asthma care may also include better partnership.

Chapter Summary

Asthma care is not standing still.

That is the central message of this chapter.

Progress has occurred.

More progress may come.

And patients should know that.

Not as hype.

But as perspective.

And as reason for grounded hope.

Action Plan

- Stay open to continued learning about asthma care.
- If asthma has been difficult to control, ask whether newer approaches deserve discussion.
- Do not assume current limitations define future possibilities.
- Stay engaged rather than drifting into resignation.
- Carry forward one important idea: grounded hope matters.

Transition to Chapter 18

We have looked at the future of asthma care. Now we come to perhaps the most practical question of all:

How do you live well with asthma over the long term?

That is where we turn next.

CHAPTER 18: Living Well with Asthma for the Long Term

We have covered a great deal in this book.

Diagnosis.

Triggers.

Treatment.

Monitoring.

Flare-ups.

Severe asthma.

And the future.

All of that matters.

But now we come to perhaps the most practical question of all:

How do you live well with asthma over the long term?

Because asthma care is not only about managing episodes.

It is about building stability.

And preserving a good life.

That is what this chapter is about.

Good Asthma Care Is Ongoing

Some patients think asthma control is something you achieve once.

And then you are done.

That is too simple.

Asthma care is often ongoing.

It involves attention.

Adjustment.

Awareness.

That is not bad news.

That is simply reality.

And once understood, it often feels less burdensome.

Because it becomes part of living.

Not something separate from life.

Stability Often Grows From Ordinary Good Habits

This may be one of the most practical lessons in the book.

Long-term stability often grows out of ordinary things done well.

Not dramatic things.

Ordinary things.

Consistency.

Awareness.

Follow-through.

These matter.

And they are often more powerful than patients realize.

Partnership Matters

Good asthma care is often strengthened by good partnership.

Communication.

Questions.

Reassessment.

Shared decision-making.

That matters.

Because patients should not feel they are carrying chronic illness alone.

Do Not Drift Away From Follow-Up

People feel better.

Life gets busy.

Follow-up slips.

Please be careful.

Drifting away from follow-up may be unwise.

Especially in chronic illness.

Because reassessment often matters.

Stay Alert to Change

Asthma may change.

Life may change.

Triggers may change.

Symptoms may change.

That is real life.

And that is why staying alert to change matters.

Not anxiously.

Thoughtfully.

There is a difference.

Thoughtful awareness is not the same as living in worry.

Living Well with Asthma

Here are some newer and advanced treatment options for asthma:

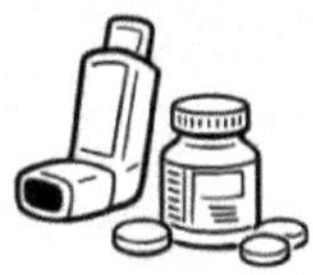

Take Medications Properly

Use your inhalers and other medications as prescribed.

↓

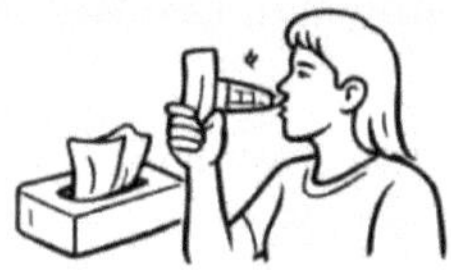

Know Your Triggers

Identify and avoid things that trigger your asthma.

↓

2. Follow Your Asthma Action Plan

Stick to your asthma management plan for best results.

↓

3. Monitor Your Symptoms

Use a peak flow meter to track your breathing.

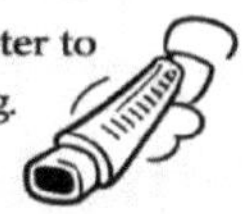

↓

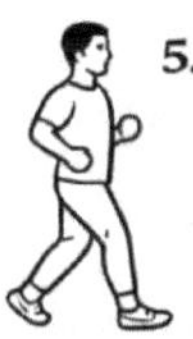

5. Stay Active Safely

Exercise regularly but within safe limits guided by your doctor.

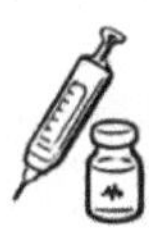

Get Vaccinated

Keep up to date with flu, pneumonia, and other vaccines.

4. Avoid Smoking

Avoid smoking and secondhand smoke exposure.

4. Keep Follow-Up Appointments

See your doctor regularly to ensure your asthma is well-managed.

By following these tips, you can manage your asthma and lead a healthy, active life.

Confidence Often Grows Through Preparedness

Confidence is not usually built by pretending nothing could go wrong.

Confidence is often built through preparedness.

Knowing what to watch.

Knowing how to respond.

Knowing what questions to ask.

That kind of confidence is durable.

And valuable.

Learn From Setbacks Without Letting Setbacks Define the Future

Flare-ups may happen.

Periods of instability may happen.

Do not let setbacks convince you all progress is lost.

That may be very wrong.

Sometimes setbacks teach.

Prompt reassessment.

Improve management.

Strengthen preparedness.

Sometimes they become part of better long-term care.

Long-Term Success Is Often Quiet

Long-term success in chronic illness is often quiet.

Not dramatic.

Fewer bad days.

More stability.

More confidence.

More life lived.

That is success.

And it should be recognized.

Monitoring Remains Part of Long-Term Success

Long-term living well does not mean abandoning monitoring.

It means integrating awareness into life wisely.

That matters.

And it supports stability.

Why This Chapter Matters

The goal of asthma care is not merely fewer symptoms.

It is living well over time.

With stability.

With confidence.

And with life preserved as fully as possible.

That is a larger goal.

And a very important one.

Doctor's Pearl

The real goal of asthma care is not merely managing episodes.

It is helping you preserve a good life over time.

Never lose sight of that.

Myth vs Fact

Myth: Long-term asthma success depends mostly on avoiding problems.

Fact: Long-term success often grows from consistency, awareness, partnership, and preparedness.

Common Mistakes to Avoid

Thinking asthma control is achieved once and then forgotten.

Drifting away from follow-up.

Letting setbacks define the future.

Confusing thoughtful monitoring with worry.

Overlooking the importance of ordinary good habits.

Red Flag Warnings

Discuss reassessment if:

- Symptoms or control begin changing
- Follow-up has lapsed
- Setbacks are becoming more frequent
- Confidence is being replaced by uncertainty
- Asthma seems intruding into life more than it should

These are important signals.

Pay attention to them.

Key Points

- Good asthma care is ongoing.
- Stability often grows from ordinary good habits.
- Partnership matters.
- Follow-up matters.
- Confidence often grows through preparedness.
- Setbacks do not have to define the future.
- The larger goal is living well.

Chapter Summary

Living well with asthma over the long term is not about perfection.

It is about building stability.

Maintaining awareness.

Staying engaged.

And preserving confidence.

That is the central lesson of this chapter.

Asthma may require attention.

But it does not have to dominate life.

Action Plan

- Think of asthma care as long-term stewardship.
- Stay consistent with the ordinary habits that support stability.
- Do not drift away from follow-up.
- Stay alert to change, but do not live in worry.
- Carry forward one important idea: living well over time is possible.

Transition to Chapter 19

As we near the close of this book, there are still important practical questions many patients commonly ask.

Questions. Misunderstandings. Everyday concerns. That is where we turn next.

CHAPTER 19: Common Questions and Myths About Asthma

Even after diagnosis.

Even after treatment.

Even after years of living with asthma.

Questions often remain.

And that is normal.

In fact, it is healthy.

Because good questions often lead to better understanding.

And better understanding often leads to better decisions.

That is why this chapter matters.

Because misunderstandings about asthma are common.

Sometimes surprisingly common.

And clearing them up may help patients think more clearly.

And live more confidently.

"If I Feel Fine, Does That Mean My Asthma Is Gone?"

This is a common question.

And an important one.

Feeling well is a good thing.

But feeling well does not necessarily mean asthma has disappeared.

Be careful with that assumption.

It may be wrong.

And sometimes risky.

Understanding the difference between feeling well and assuming the condition no longer matters is important.

"If I Only Have Symptoms Occasionally, Does Asthma Really Matter?"

Another very common question.

And a very understandable one.

Intermittent symptoms may still matter.

We discussed this earlier.

It deserves emphasis here.

Because people sometimes dismiss conditions that are not constantly intrusive.

Be careful.

Intermittent does not necessarily mean trivial.

"Will I Always Have Asthma?"

Patients ask this often.

And understandably so.

The answer may depend on the individual.

And this is an area where oversimplification helps no one.

What matters most for this book is not offering false certainty.

But emphasizing something practical:

Focus on understanding, monitoring, and good management.

That is where patients have influence.

"Should I Avoid Exercise?"

This myth deserves direct attention.

No.

Do not assume that.

Exercise should not automatically be placed on an avoidance list simply because someone has asthma.

That assumption may do harm.

Be careful with it.

"If I Need More Treatment, Does That Mean I Am Getting Worse?"

Another misconception.

And an important one.

Not necessarily.

Please do not assume that.

Treatment decisions may reflect many considerations.

And assumptions can mislead.

Questions should lead to discussion.

Not discouragement.

"Is Asthma Mostly Psychological?"

I want to answer this clearly.

No.

Asthma is a real medical condition.

That should not be muddied.

Ever.

Can stress affect symptoms or symptom experience?

Sometimes it may.

But do not confuse that with claiming asthma is "just psychological."

That is false.

And unhelpful.

"Should I Be Afraid of the Future?"

This is often not asked aloud.

But many patients carry it quietly.

So I want to address it.

No.

Do not let fear become your organizing principle.

Be thoughtful.

Be prepared.

Stay engaged.

But do not let fear quietly become the center of the story.

Myths Often Persist Because They Sound Simple

Myths often survive because they offer simple explanations.

But simple explanations are not always true explanations.

Be cautious with simplistic thinking.

In medicine.

And in life.

That caution serves people well.

Good Questions Improve Care

I want patients to feel encouraged to ask.

Not embarrassed to ask.

Not reluctant to ask.

Encouraged.

Questions improve care.

Always.

And patients should remember that.

Why This Chapter Matters

Misunderstandings can quietly affect decisions.

And decisions matter.

This chapter is about clearing away confusion.

And reinforcing practical truths.

Doctor's Pearl

One of the healthiest habits a patient can develop is this:

Question assumptions.

Especially simple assumptions.

That habit often protects people from mistakes.

Myth vs Fact

Myth: Asthma is simple, obvious, and easy to understand once diagnosed.

Fact: Questions and misconceptions are common, and continuing to ask good questions matters.

Common Mistakes to Avoid

Assuming feeling well means asthma has disappeared.

Assuming intermittent symptoms do not matter.

Assuming exercise should be avoided.

Assuming more treatment automatically means failure.

Letting myths replace thoughtful understanding.

Red Flag Warnings

Reopen discussion if:

- You are making decisions based on assumptions you have never questioned
- Fear is quietly shaping major decisions
- Confusion about asthma remains unresolved
- Myths or misinformation are influencing choices

These are excellent reasons to revisit questions.

Key Points

- Questions about asthma are normal.
- Feeling well does not necessarily mean asthma has disappeared.
- Intermittent symptoms may still matter.
- Exercise should not automatically be avoided.
- Asthma is a real medical condition, not "just psychological."
- Myths can mislead.
- Good questions improve care.

Chapter Summary

Questions and misconceptions about asthma are common.

That is the central lesson of this chapter.

Do not let myths quietly shape decisions.

Question assumptions.

Ask good questions.

And seek thoughtful understanding.

That matters.

Action Plan

- Identify one asthma belief or assumption you may never have questioned.
- Revisit whether it deserves reconsideration.
- Write down unanswered questions you still have.
- Do not let myths or fear quietly guide important decisions.
- Carry forward one important idea: good questions improve care.

Transition to Chapter 20

We have covered science.

Symptoms.

Treatment.

Setbacks.

Possibility.

And long-term living.

Now we come to the final question:

What should you carry forward from all of this?

That is where we turn next.

CHAPTER 20: Living With Asthma, Living Beyond Asthma

We have covered a great deal together.

What asthma is.

What may cause it.

How it is recognized.

How it is diagnosed.

How it is treated.

How to monitor it.

How to think about flare-ups.

How to live actively.

How to think about severe asthma.

How to think about possibility.

And how to live well over time.

That has been the journey of this book.

And now we come to the final question:

What should you carry forward from all of this?

I hope it is this:

Perspective.

Confidence.

And a wider understanding of what asthma does, and does not, have to mean.

Because the final chapter of a book should not merely repeat information.

It should help clarify what matters most.

That is what I hope this chapter does.

Asthma May Require Attention, But It Need Not Define You

A diagnosis describes a medical condition.

It does not define a human being.

Never confuse the two.

You are more than a diagnosis.

Always.

That matters.

And it is worth saying plainly.

Do Not Let Asthma Quietly Become the Center of the Story

Be careful what role you allow illness to assume in your inner life.

Illness may require attention.

Sometimes significant attention.

But attention is not identity.

Do not let those become confused.

That distinction matters greatly.

Carry Forward Understanding, Not Fear

If there is one emotional lesson I hope readers carry from this book, it is this:

Replace unnecessary fear with informed understanding.

Fear narrows.

Understanding clarifies.

Fear may make life smaller.

Understanding may restore perspective.

That matters.

Carry Forward Preparedness, Not Hypervigilance

There is a difference.

A very important difference.

Preparedness is wise.

Hypervigilance is exhausting.

Do not confuse them.

Carry forward preparedness.

Let go of unnecessary over-monitoring driven by fear.

That is not the same as good care.

Carry Forward Questions

Good patients are often thoughtful questioners.

And I hope this book has encouraged that.

Keep asking questions.

Keep staying engaged.

Keep resisting passive resignation.

That matters.

Carry Forward Perspective

This may be the heart of the chapter.

Perspective.

Because chronic illness can distort perspective.

Symptoms can feel bigger than life.

Fear can feel bigger than possibility.

Setbacks can feel bigger than progress.

Be careful.

Perspective matters.

And sometimes protecting perspective is part of protecting health.

Progress Matters

Do not forget this.

We discussed progress in asthma care.

It matters.

Carry that forward too.

Do not quietly assume the future is closed.

It is not.

Possibility matters.

Living Beyond Asthma Does Not Mean Pretending Asthma Does Not Exist

This is important balance.

I am not advocating denial.

Living beyond asthma does not mean ignoring asthma.

It means refusing to let asthma define the boundaries of your identity or possibilities unnecessarily.

That is something much wiser.

And much healthier.

What I Hope You Carry Forward Most

If I had to reduce this entire book to a few thoughts, perhaps it would be these:

Understand your condition.

Ask questions.

Stay engaged.

Respect symptoms.

Use treatment thoughtfully.

Do not accept poor control too easily.

Do not let fear quietly shrink life.

And do not let a diagnosis define you.

Those are not small things.

Those are very large things.

And I hope they stay with you.

Why This Chapter Matters

Information alone is not enough.

Readers should leave a book carrying something more than facts.

They should leave carrying perspective.

And I hope this chapter offers that.

Doctor's Pearl

A diagnosis may require attention.

But it should never be allowed to quietly become the definition of who you are.

Never forget that.

Myth vs Fact

Myth: Living well with asthma means simply learning to live within the limits asthma imposes.

Fact: Thoughtful asthma care is often about preserving possibility, not surrendering to unnecessary limitation.

Common Mistakes to Avoid

Letting fear quietly become the center of the story.

Confusing preparedness with hypervigilance.

Letting setbacks distort perspective.

Allowing a diagnosis to become identity.

Assuming chronic illness automatically means a smaller life.

Red Flag Warnings

Reopen discussion if:

- Fear is quietly dominating your decisions
- You have accepted limitations you have never questioned
- Discouragement has become resignation
- Asthma feels as though it is defining too much of your life

These are important signals worth taking seriously.

Key Points

- Asthma may require attention, but it need not define you.
- Carry forward understanding, not fear.
- Carry forward preparedness, not hypervigilance.

- Keep asking questions.
- Protect perspective.
- Do not let a diagnosis define identity or possibility.
- Living beyond asthma is about preserving a full life.

Chapter Summary

Asthma is real.

It deserves attention.

Thoughtful care.

Respect.

But it does not have to define the limits of your life.

That is the central message of this chapter.

Carry forward understanding.

Carry forward perspective.

Carry forward confidence.

And above all, do not let a diagnosis become smaller than the life that holds it.

Action Plan

- Reflect on whether fear has shaped any limits you may want to reconsider.
- Carry forward the habits of thoughtful engagement this book has emphasized.
- Protect perspective.

- Refuse to let a diagnosis quietly define identity.
- Carry forward one important idea: asthma may require attention, but it need not define your life.

Final Thought

If this book has helped you understand asthma more clearly, ask better questions, feel less afraid, or feel more hopeful, then it has served its purpose.

And I would be grateful for that.

APPENDIX A: Personal Asthma Action Plan Worksheet

Use this worksheet to organize important information about your asthma care.

Discuss and complete it with your physician if appropriate.

My Asthma Medicines

Daily medicines I take:

____

____

Quick-relief medicine:

____

My Possible Triggers

Possible triggers I have noticed:

____

____

____

Signs My Asthma May Be Worsening

Symptoms I want to watch for:

____

____

What I Will Do If Symptoms Worsen

Steps I plan to take:

____

____

Important Contact Information

My physician:

____

Phone:

____

Emergency contact:

____

This worksheet is meant to support preparation, not replace medical advice.

APPENDIX B: Questions to Ask Your Doctor About Asthma

Bring these questions to your next visit if helpful.

About My Diagnosis

- How certain is my diagnosis?
- Should any additional testing be considered?
- Are there other conditions that may also be contributing?

About My Treatment

- Why am I taking each medicine?
- Is my inhaler technique correct?
- Are there side effects I should understand?

About My Asthma Control

- Is my asthma well controlled?
- Could control be improved?
- What warning signs should I watch for?

About Flare-Ups and Emergencies

- Do I need a written asthma action plan?
- When should I seek urgent help?
- What should I do if symptoms worsen unexpectedly?

About the Future

- Are there additional treatment options I should know about?
- Should I ever consider specialist evaluation?

Good questions improve care.

Bring them.

Ask them.

Use them.

APPENDIX C: A 30-Day Asthma Awareness and Stability Plan

Week 1

Observe.

Pay attention to symptoms.

Notice patterns.

Notice possible triggers.

Write things down.

Week 2

Review.

Review medicines.

Review inhaler technique.

Review whether questions remain unanswered.

Week 3

Strengthen.

Address one trigger more thoughtfully.

Revisit activity goals.

Improve one daily habit that may support stability.

Week 4

Plan.

Review what you have learned.

Write down ongoing questions.

Think about long-term habits that support good asthma care.

Carry those forward.

Final Note to Readers

Asthma management is rarely about perfection.

It is often about awareness.

Preparedness.

Consistency.

And thoughtful partnership.

That is what I hope this book has supported.

Thank You and Please Review the Book

Thank you for taking the time to read this book. I sincerely hope it has helped you understand your health a little more clearly and has given you practical, everyday steps you can follow with confidence. If you found this book helpful, **I would truly appreciate it if you could leave a brief and honest review.** Even a few lines sharing your experience can make a meaningful difference. Your feedback helps other readers find reliable, trustworthy health information and supports them in making better decisions for themselves and their families.

Warm regards,

Dr Prabhat Das

Continue your Healthcare Journey

Good health is a journey, not a single step. It is not achieved in one day or with one book. That is why I created the "Better Health with Dr Das" series, with each book addressing a different common condition. If you would like easy, practical guidance on other everyday health concerns, you may wish to explore the rest of books in this series.

Books in this series:

- Better Health starts Here: A Doctor's Guide to Staying Healthy After 40
- A Doctor's Easy Guide to Understanding & Managing OBESITY
- Doctor, What DIET Is Best for Me?
- Doctor, Why Can't I Lose Weight? A Doctor's Guide to safe & Sustainable Weight Loss)
- A Doctor's Easy Guide to GLP-1 for Obesity
- A Doctor's Easy Guide to Understanding & Managing HIGH BLOOD PRESSURE
- A Doctor's Guide to Living Well With DIABETES
- A Doctor's Guide to Understanding & Managing THYROID DISEASES
- A Doctor's Guide to Understanding & Managing HIGH CHOLESTEROL
- A Doctor's Practical Guide to HEART HEALTH After 40: How to Protect Your Heart & Live Longer
- A Doctor's Guide to Healing & Reversing FATTY LIVER DISEASE: Simple, Natural & Science-Based Steps to Reduce Liver Fat and Prevent Complications

- Control Your ACID REFLUX, HEARTBURN & GERD: A Doctor's Practical Guide that Works
- Live Comfortably with IRRITABLE BOWEL SYNDROME: A Doctor's Practical Guide to Understanding & Managing IBS
- A Doctor's Practical Guide to Understanding & Managing GALLBLADDER STONES & OTHER PROBLEMS
- Take Control of COPD: A Doctor's Practical Guide to Better Breathing
- Living Better with ASTHMA: A Doctor's Practical Guide to Asthma Control
- SLEEP APNEA & SNORING: A Doctor's Practical Guide to Better Sleep & Better Health
- KIDNEY STONES: A Doctor's Practical Guide to Prevention & Care
- Protect Your KIDNEYS: A Doctor's Practical Guide to Kidney Health & Prevention
- PROSTATE HEALTH After 40: A Doctor's Practical Guide to Early Detection & Care
- ARTHRITIS: A Doctor's Practical Guide to Pain Control & Mobility
- A Doctor's Practical Guide to Fixing BACK PAIN Step by Step
- A Doctor's Practical Guide to Understanding & Managing GOUT & URIC ACID and Preventing Complications
- HEALTHY SKIN & COMMON SKIN PROBLEMS: A Doctor's Practical Guide to Skin Care
- DEMENTIA & MEMORY LOSS: A Doctor's Practical Guide to Prevention & Management
- Doctor, Why Am I TIRED All The Time? Fixing Fatigue & Getting Your Energy Back

9 781971 672465

Printed by Libri Plureos GmbH in Hamburg,
Germany